T0128289

"Alison writes from her heart and inspires her readers to live well, to live healthy and to live with hope. I'm so thankful for the encouragement and stepping stones that she shares to live well so I am better able to give more of myself to others."

"A delightful read and one I'll be sharing with friends and family."

— Donna Mitchell

"*Don't Let What if? Ruin What Is*, is a full spectrum experience touching on all aspects of life. With a mix of passion, authenticity, compassion and friendship, Alison takes your hand and brings you on a journey through her life experience and reveals what led her to freedom from anxiety and control and provided her with a lasting peace. Her faith, personal stories and practical tips offer guidance and declare hope for the future, healing and freedom. May you find the one who can bring peace to your soul in these pages!"

— Jan Pritchard

Don't Let
What if?
Ruin
What Is

A Mom's Guide to Worry
Less and Live More

ALISON BROWN

WESTBOW
PRESS®
A DIVISION OF THOMAS NELSON
& ZONDERVAN

This book is a work of non-fiction. Unless otherwise noted, the author and the publisher make no explicit guarantees as to the accuracy of the information contained in this book and in some cases, names of people and places have been altered to protect their privacy.

WestBow Press books may be ordered through booksellers or by contacting:

WestBow Press
A Division of Thomas Nelson & Zondervan
1663 Liberty Drive
Bloomington, IN 47403
www.westbowpress.com
844-714-3454

Because of the dynamic nature of the Internet, any web addresses or links contained in this book may have changed since publication and may no longer be valid. The views expressed in this work are solely those of the author and do not necessarily reflect the views of the publisher, and the publisher hereby disclaims any responsibility for them.

Any people depicted in stock imagery provided by Getty Images are models, and such images are being used for illustrative purposes only. Certain stock imagery © Getty Images.

Scripture taken from the New King James Version®. Copyright © 1982 by Thomas Nelson. Used by permission. All rights reserved.

ISBN: 978-1-6642-9220-8 (sc)
ISBN: 978-1-6642-9221-5 (hc)
ISBN: 978-1-6642-9219-2 (e)

Library of Congress Control Number: 2023902642

Print information available on the last page.

WestBow Press rev. date: 02/21/2023

Contents

Dedication

To my Heavenly Father, who has set me free from worry and given me eternal life in Christ Jesus. Thank you for your unconditional love and the firm foundation.

To my dad, whose death gave me a new life and whose words of wisdom are the reason I write. I love you and miss you every day, but I am comforted to know we will see each other again.

And, to anyone who has lost sleep, peace, and joy because of worry and wondered if they could ever live free, God finished this work so you could finish working and rest in the freedom only he can offer.

"Therefore, do not worry about tomorrow,
for tomorrow will worry about itself."
Mathew 6:34

Foreword

Over the course of my life, I have often pondered the imbalanced scales of difficult things that people face in their lives. For example, while one family is experiencing good health, joy in relationships, as well as success in business, finances, and other achievements, another battles chronic or terminal illness, mental health, loss, trauma, and financial instability. These events may happen in rapid succession, or they may occur all at once. While I don't have an answer why things happen this way, I have discovered in my life that it is possible for great pain to bring forth wisdom and understanding that may not have surfaced without it.

You may have heard the phrase, "Smooth seas never made a skilled sailor." The statement implies that if the waters are calm, a sailor will never use the knowledge gained while training practically. Their skill level needs a chance to develop. When things are smooth and easy, they miss out on the opportunity to work out the kinks and build confidence as they test out what works and what doesn't.

If this statement is true of life, then those around us who appear to be on stormy seas frequently in their personal lives are developing skills that the rest of us could stand to learn from. Alison is one of these people. If you haven't hit a stormy sea yet, life almost certainly guarantees it will come at some point, and when it does, you will surely want some wisdom to lean on, and I believe Alison has a great deal of it to share with us.

Over the last year, I have heard Alison's story about experiences, present difficulties, and plans as her mentor during a course we provide within our organization. Even though I had some prior knowledge of the stories found in the pages of this book, I found myself in awe of the size and weight of the situations and events she has experienced over the course of her life as I read. This caused me to lean in and search for the wisdom I could gather from her experience.

If I could sum up what I found in one statement, it would be this: "What I walk through in this life matters, but how I respond to it matters even more." Difficult circumstances make it hard to remain present and cause us to feel out of control. Considering this, we grip the reins of our lives tighter until we are white knuckling it through life with gritted teeth, just hoping to survive or find various ways of seeking comfort and escape.

Alison, gently and yet with determination, shares with us that there is another way to approach life's challenges. In this book, you will discover that it is possible to not only survive life's challenges but also thrive during them and experience peace and health. You will receive practical tips for caring for yourself both mentally and physically. You will learn to look for the gifts hidden deep within the storms of life and discover the Creator who holds all things together and can sustain you when the seas are rough. As Alison pours out many experiences from her life and what she's learned in and through them, you find you are not alone in the battle and that it is possible to set down the burden of anxiety and choose to pick up peace and rest.

I have had the opportunity this year to really listen and hear Alison's heart for you, the reader. I know how much she longs for you to know that you are not alone and there is hope. Alison is a delight and joy to be around. Her sensitive heart conveys a deep care for others, and I hope you can feel just how much she believes in you. More than this, I hope you can see just how powerfully she has experienced the presence of God in her life and how her faith is the key to it all.

This was a faith forged in the fire; it did not come to her easily. Her stormy seas were so rough that she needed to rely on something bigger than herself to get through it all. She chose God. With every difficulty, her faith has been strengthened as she experiences how He gets her through it. If you have not met God in this way, I know Alison would tell you He is absolutely worth getting to know and that He is ready, willing, and able to get your boat through the storm because He loves you. If you are tired and what you have been doing to get by doesn't seem to work, I hope that through these pages you will come face to face with the source of true rest and experience a peace greater than anything you've ever known.

Jan Pritchard
Discipleship Counselor
Crossways to Life

If your pile is too big,
stop trying to hold it up;
set it down instead.

Introduction

The things we carry...

A few years ago, I came across an eye-opening piece of artwork. I was looking for cement garden art, and I was scrolling and found a lifelike cement-sculpture mom standing hunched over on a sidewalk. I couldn't stop staring at it. It was the visual definition of a truth bomb.

This exhausted sculpture mom carried her child in one arm and wore a giant pile of household objects stacked up almost sky high on her back. She slouched forward under the weight of the washer, vacuum cleaner, pots, pans, and more. Of course, in true mom fashion, she still kept it all up—the cement certainly helped.

A team of artists in Spain had perfectly depicted what so many moms, myself included, can relate to. They called their masterpiece *The Weight on a Mother's Shoulders.*

It was as if someone had held up a mirror right in front of me and showed me what I looked like. Seeing my reflection was revelatory. Suddenly, I understood why I felt so exhausted. It all made perfect sense. I was trying to hold it all up. That was the first problem. The second one was that I wasn't made of cement.

I let my mind wander as I fixed my gaze on the image in front of me. I thought of the many questions I would ask this statue mom if she were real: How is your back feeling? How long can you hold it all up? How long can you live your life crouched under the weight of all these things you're carrying? Will you ever stop trying so hard to keep it all together? What will happen to not only your back but also your emotional and mental state when someone comes along and adds to that already impossible-to-hold-up pile? With enough weight on it, even the strongest of cement will crumble.

As I asked these questions, I knew I was really asking them to myself. I could completely relate to this very overwhelmed, almost-falling-over, busy mom, and I knew so many other moms who could, too.

She was real. I was her but without the cement. I had just recently collapsed under the weight of the millions of things I was trying so hard to carry (more on that soon), and when I did, I almost couldn't get back up.

Contrary to what the world may think of us moms—that we are superhero, got-it-all-together, multi-tasking miracle workers—even moms can't hold it all up.

Often, we are the cement that holds it all together. Without us, it really can all come crashing down, and sometimes, despite our best efforts, it does anyway; ourselves included.

When a mom falls down, it's rare for someone to be there to help her back up. It's almost always she who must stand herself back up, dust herself off, and carry on again. She gets up because she has to. She moves on to the next job without even being able to care for the wounds inflicted by her fall. Survival mode sets in, and she soldiers on.

It's not even the crash that impacts moms the most; it's the trying to keep it all from crashing that has the biggest impact. Trying to hold it all up is exhausting. It spreads moms thin and doesn't allow them to be good for anyone who needs and loves them.

The crash would actually be a good thing. For me, it was. After everything came smashing down around me, myself included, I could carefully re-evaluate what I even wanted to pick back up.

Once I survived the fall, I got up lighter and could move

forward with a freedom I couldn't keep to myself. It was too liberating to hide. Discovering there was a happier and lighter way to be a mom was like getting a dishwasher after years of handwashing them—glorious!

Today, if this mom statue was real, I would help her throw that pile down without her experiencing one worry or shred of guilt for having done so. All that would remain is that sweet little one in her arms for her to simply enjoy and a free hand so she could care for herself, too, which is equally important. And I would argue *even more important.*

If you're this statue mom, it's time for you to lighten that load and enjoy the little one(s), or bigger ones, that made you mom in the first place, without all the junk on your back. It's time to let go of all the things weighing you down and be a mom without all the stuff.

This sculpture is a shocking depiction of the way things are for too many moms right now, at this very moment. The artists nailed it. The cement mom represents moms everywhere, and the artists simply held up a mirror to show the world what a mom really looks like. Not all moms, but certainly many, are falling under the weight of the countless demands, duties, tasks, roles, and giant expectations.

Too many are exhausting themselves to ensure their ducks are in a row. With a smile on their face, and a rosy Instagram picture, they appear to be doing very well, but under the surface, the only thing in a row is the mile long list of to-dos that keeps accumulating and the overwhelm that comes from the stress of trying to get it all done.

Their ducks are flying in ten different directions, and they're chasing them while they're under slept, over caffeinated, and stressed out. They smile over it. They clean over it. They shop over it. They cover it all up like a good age-defying makeup. But under the surface, they are suffering. Moms are suffering. Bit by bit, they not only lose themselves amidst it all, but they also lose their joy.

Their peace lasts just a few minutes as they sit and sip a glass of wine or tea at the end of the day and indulge in their favorite snack. If they're lucky enough to have no external interruptions, like the four-year-old needing to be tucked in again, for the third time, or the nine-year-old needing food, or the teenager blaring his or her music, their minds do an excellent job of stealing that peace all on their very own. They list to-dos. They make mental notes of what they did wrong today. They feel guilty about it. They beat themselves up over it, and then, the subject I can't wait to broach, they worry themselves into an absolute state.

Instead of sleeping, they ruminate about all the things that could go wrong. They stack them up sky high. They worry that they're doing it all wrong. They worry about the future, and they trail off into a tangent of what could go wrong right now.

Under the smile and the "I'm fine," their joy is fleeting. Despite their best attempts, for many, their excitement for motherhood left the house right around the same time the two-year-old started throwing temper tantrums or, maybe even sooner, when junior never slept long enough for anyone to feel sane.

What's worse is they feel guilty and conflicted admitting how they really feel about motherhood because they love their children to the depths of their souls and wouldn't trade them for anything. They also know or know of women who would do anything to be mom, so they wouldn't dare say a word of this out loud. And yet, they long for peace and happiness, but they live with this ongoing inner conflict they say nothing about.

Sure, there are moments, sometimes even days and seasons, of happiness and joy, but they never seem to last. The reality of laundry piles, meeting "I wants," and catering to the constant demands always seems to scare them away.

It's short lived and yet so is the time they get with their kids, so they swallow the good with the not so good and soldier on, knowing all of this is gone in literally the blink of an eye. The kids grow up, and mom's job, though never done, will look much different, and deep in their souls, they have this awareness that they will probably even miss these very busy days.

So, they keep going and keep trying to hold their exhausting giant pile up. They've accepted the cost of motherhood without even knowing that there doesn't have to be one. There honestly is a better way to live.

They don't have to carry so many things—the kids, the laundry, the meals, the vacuum cleaner, the broom, the backpacks, the snack bags, the laptop, the keys, the purse, the groceries, the schedule, and the millions of toys and clothes that accumulate on the floors daily.

Not to mention—the planning of birthday parties, Christmas's, family vacations, and, of course, the packing for such events, and then the dreaded unpacking and clean up after it's all over.

These tangibles are all heavy, but I would argue they are light compared to the figurative things so many moms choose to carry. Let's add some more reality to this very real and extremely full pile. Throw on self doubt, the desire for perfection, the guilt, the stress of racing to get the endless tasks of mom completed, the constant feelings of failure that come with dropping one of the many balls being juggled, the fear of getting it all wrong. I can't even recount how many times I've asked myself, *Am I messing them up forever?* And, of course, the list of what ifs?

The exhausting, often-irrational, aggravating, sleep-robbing rabbit hole of *What if this happens?* that never stops nagging, much like an unrelenting child who asks for another cookie again and again and again, although you've said no for what feels like the millionth time already.

The heaviness that comes from trying to keep it all together and worrying *what if* every second of my day made me collapse, and this crash was literally the wake up that I needed. The things I was trying to hold up, along with the worrying I was doing, were stealing my peace, joy, sleep, and the mom I wanted to be for my children. It holds us all back from living the lives we deserve to live—the life that God intended when he made us moms.

Thankfully, my crash, in the form of an epic mommy meltdown, made me realize that I've got some unpacking to do, some self care to focus on, some heavy stuff to throw away, and above all, some worrying to stop; worrying I didn't even realize I was doing.

This mom pile that so many moms think they should be able to hold up can actually be set down. Being a mom doesn't have to look like the statue. To discover your freedom, you'll need to first have a solid look at what has been trapping you. For me, that was the habit of worry.

Now, I should interrupt for a second with a disclaimer that I am a God-loving mom to three boys, a fitness and nutrition expert, and an online mom-tribe entrepreneur. I am not a worry expert—although I could win some prizes for the amount of worrying I've done over the years.

The advice in the coming pages is from a professional worrier who's been in remission for a few years with some minor relapses here and there. I've got a story to share and some tools to give you to help you overcome your struggles.

As I've lightened my load, I've been able to help countless other moms lighten theirs as well and not just that, but also regain their life in the process. In the coming pages, it is entirely possible that along with setting worry down, I may convince you to trust God more, possibly take up exercise and eating healthy, and lighten your load a little by setting a few things down you weren't even aware you were carrying. I may even convince you that your needs and wants are just as important as your children's, and that you need to be a priority to be healthy for everyone who needs and loves you. If any of the above occurs, then my mission will have been accomplished.

I am sharing my story, hoping to help you discover yours doesn't have to be one where worry wins. My personal journey has been one with near deaths of my son, husband, and myself, the tragic loss of a friend, the death of my dad to ALS, a plane crash, a job loss at seven months pregnant with two kids, a few car accidents, and some traumatic childhood challenges to heal from.

I've got a million valid reasons to worry, but I choose to live my life instead. I'll share my story in the coming pages with the hope it will encourage you and bring awareness to your worrying habits so you, too, can set them down and start living a happier, healthier, more peace-filled life. *What if?* doesn't have to steal what is from this moment forward. It's time to turn the page.

I never used to worry, but
then I became a mom.

CHAPTER 1

Burn the Habit Before It Burns You

Some people bite their nails, others swear or say "um" or "like" a lot, some have a physical gesture they do repeatedly, and some people worry.

It's a habit. That's what worrying is, or I should say that's what it becomes. Like anything, the more you do it, the better you get at it. With practice and repetition, it slowly seeps into the default setting of your mind and becomes a part of the inner fabric of your being.

Eventually, it's just automatic and feels so natural that you don't even have to be conscious of doing it to do it. Your mind can autopilot into a tangent of *what if* without even being aware of what is happening.

Despite having learned how to control it, I still jump off a cliff now and then even when we aren't anywhere near one. The good news is that I have to let myself go there, as opposed to doing it automatically.

Now I have the awareness of the choice I'm making and actually have to give myself permission to do it. This is incredible progress. Honestly, I've come so far from the professional worrier I once was. But before I celebrate my victory, let's back up a little to a time before I even knew this was something I walked around carrying.

There are several moments that stand out for me as I reflect on my worrying habit. One of them is when I discovered I was pregnant. I was a functional worrier until that magical moment I got to actually see the baby I was housing. Then I became a severely dysfunctional one.

Here's what I mean; the minute I saw that precious, little human inside my belly on the ultrasound monitor, with his teeny, little hands and feet and oddly shaped large but precious head, was the same minute my worrying habit reared its ugly head and started spiraling out of control. I know the hormone roller coaster I was riding contributed to the problem. Couple that with the realization that another human fully depended on me for his very survival, and suddenly, I felt this massive pressure. It was as if a giant weight was thrown onto my back.

Maybe you can relate? I had this baby's life depending on me, and I really didn't want to mess anything up. I needed to get it all right. There was absolutely no margin for error. I'm also a recovering perfectionist, so when I tell you no margin, I mean no margin.

The ultrasound was supposed to be this glorious moment where I got a sneak peek at the miracle I housed, and though it was that, it was also a terrifying moment because it made everything so real for me and with that came worry.

I worried about what I ate, what I didn't eat, what I did, what I didn't do, what vitamins were safe, whether I should dye my hair, what cleaning products were safe, if listeria was in my cantaloupe, and on and on, I worried.

I stressed about tiny stuff and far-fetched big stuff too, and then I Googled it all, which gave me a brand-new list of things to worry about. Every symptom, ache, pain, and twinge I had during my pregnancy became cause for concern. I feared miscarrying, or the baby not being healthy, or the birth being traumatic. I pondered everything you might think of and even the things you can't imagine.

I literally spent countless nights reading what-to-expect books, watching baby shows, and fearing something awful would happen that I didn't expect at all. I thought of every worst-case scenario and almost every impossible one, too.

If I continued to list all the what ifs I let my mind fester on and Googled while my first baby boy was growing in my belly, you'd either think I was totally off my rocker, or the familiarity would mean we both have some work to do.

Letting my mind wander way beyond the realm of logic became a well-practiced habit for me. I was good at it. So good it became natural, and eventually, I didn't even have to let myself go there to go there. I did it automatically. What's worse is that I didn't even know I was doing it. It became so natural that I was no longer aware it was even happening.

Despite it all sounding so insane in hindsight, at the time, it was all very real and even rational because I worried in disguise. I told myself I was "researching," "educating myself," and "staying on top of all the details I needed to know during the pregnancy," but I was trying to control something I had no control over.

Education disguised my worrying habit for a little while. Somehow, I felt more in control when I knew of every possible worst-case scenario—or at least that's what I told myself.

That's oddly what worry is—a way to try to control when we are out of control entirely. Instead of being able to relax, let it all go, and trust that it will work out, we worry it won't, and though the logic seems faulty, this gives the illusion of control over a situation that is completely out of our hands.

Looking back, I am sick to think of all the time and sleep I wasted stressing over things that never even happened. Some nights, I would wake up my husband, Graham, and say things like, "What if the baby doesn't make it?" or, "What if the baby comes too early?" or, "What if I die giving birth? That can happen, you know." He would always say the same thing, "Whatever happens, we will deal with it; now go back to sleep."

Honestly, if I could rewind my life, I would tell that younger, pregnant, over-informed me to listen to my husband and go to sleep. The baby will do a fine job of interrupting your slumber all on his own.

Knowing me, though, I probably wouldn't have listened, anyway. It honestly took a mommy meltdown to finally open my ears and wake me up to the fact that I was carrying stuff I never even needed to pick up to begin with.

With each pregnancy and each new baby boy (I have three), the worrying culminated. And like anything that culminates, one summer day, it all came to an ugly, explosive head.

The weight of worry, the overwhelm that comes with caring for two toddlers and a newborn baby, all the stuff us moms throw onto our backs and try hard to prop up, combined with the lack of caring for myself amidst it all, landed me on the floor in my bathroom in a pool of my exhausted tears.

I've relayed this meltdown to thousands of moms over the years to share with them what can happen when we try to carry more than we can carry.

I want moms to know that it's okay to set some things down. I know firsthand the cost of not doing that. I also want moms to know that asking for help is the best thing you can do for yourself and your loved ones. It's good to ask for help. It doesn't make you weak or mean that you're incapable; it means you are brave and wise. It means you know your limitations and are human. I certainly wish I would have asked for help instead of trying to do it all myself.

I'll share my story with you with the same intentions and the hope that it will help you re-evaluate all the things you may be carrying that you can set down. Otherwise, like they did for me, they could all come crashing down instead.

On the day of this monumental crash, I was extra sleep

deprived. I had been going a few months on little to no sleep. Zachary, my youngest, had just recovered from pneumonia and was not sleeping well, which left me extra tired all the time. Extra tired for me usually left me short-tempered with Andrew and Levi and extra emotional. Lack of sleep, in combination with the lie that I needed to set my needs aside and look after everyone else's instead, was a recipe for disaster.

I remember the exact time of this meltdown because I was counting the minutes until Graham returned home from work to help take some of the load I was carrying. It was 4 p.m., and despite only having one more hour until he was home, I dreaded 4 p.m. every single day. For some reason, 4 p.m. felt like the hour that all chaos was breaking loose in my home. This seemed to be the hour that my kids misbehaved the most, and I almost always lost my cool. Today, though, I would lose my mind as well.

All three of my children were hungry, which meant blood sugar was at an all-time low, and this always makes them extra wild. I was doing my best to clean and cook dinner and cater to every call. I got them drinks and a small snack to tie them over until dinner was ready and was trying to entertain them while I held Zachary, who, since his birth, never wanted down and only wanted his mom.

I distinctly remember the thought crossing my mind that I just wanted to sleep for days, but instead of taking a five-minute break like I probably should have, I filled up a fourth cup of cold coffee, guzzled it down like a thirsty child, and continued to cook with the baby on my hip and an exhausted soul.

It wasn't one distinct incident or moment that set me off; it was a series of moments that escalated into a giant explosion. As I recall, my oldest son, Andrew, who was five at the time, was bothering my middle son, Levi, who was three; this is a common occurrence in our home—brotherly love. It drives me bananas on a good day. Levi was dishing it out just as much. The newest addition to our family, baby Zachary, was crying because he needed to be fed, and I was racing to do everything for everyone all at the same time, like most moms do.

Someone spilled a cup of water, someone threw food across the table, the baby cried harder, and I raced to get him fed, which forced me to sit down and nurse him while my food boiled over and the other two fought.

The tipping point, though, was Andrew and Levi's squabble escalated into a physical fight, a big one. One I had been warned by fellow boy moms about but had yet to witness until now. Today was not the day for me to break it up calmly. Today I yelled. I yelled and yelled until it became an out-of-control scream. It was as if my soul unleashed years of frustration all at once. I don't recall the words that came out of my mouth, but I recall the stunned look on Andrew's and Levi's faces.

They were suddenly silent with their eyes wide open. Fear took over their precious faces, and tears came down mine like a flood that I couldn't hold back. The dam was broken. I had somehow released a raging river, and there was no stopping it now. I angrily set Zachary in the middle of the living room, turned the stove off, and then forcefully picked Andrew up and literally threw him into his room. I slammed the door so hard I almost broke it. Then I grabbed Levi and threw him on a step for a timeout. I had never been so loud or so rough with my children or so out of control of my emotions and actions. Every frustration came raging out of me and unleashed a beast in our home at that moment.

I carried Zachary to the bathroom and locked the door. With a crying and no doubt terrified baby in my arms, I collapsed onto the floor and called my husband's cell. I am so thankful I even had someone I could call because I honestly don't even want to know what would have happened had he not been there. I was irrational and enraged and exhausted all at the same time.

As the phone rang, I prayed he would answer it and be able to leave work early. Running our own business has a lot of demands, and he can't always leave on a whim. By now, I could hear my traumatized boys outside my bathroom door crying and calling for me, begging me to come out.

Andrew is an extremely empathetic, beautifully sensitive boy, and I could hear him telling me he loves me and that he is sorry. Levi chimed in and sweetly whispered, "Sorry, mommy." I can imagine my uncontrollable, desperate sobs sounded horrible to them. I felt guilty for what they had just experienced and reassured them I would be out soon. I promised them that everything was okay, even though I wasn't sure myself that it was. Children are smart. I know they knew I was lying.

Hearing Graham's voice on the phone immediately calmed me down. Graham always has a way of doing that. It's one of the many things I love about him. I begged him to come home and explained that I needed his help. I'm sure he could hear it in my voice, despite me trying to hide it.

I hated needing help, and it was so hard for me to ask for it, but I knew it was good that I called him. A small sense of relief came over me, knowing he could leave work early and save his kids from their mom. Despite the relief, I equally felt horrible that they even needed saving.

While he was on his way, I sat on the cold bathroom floor in a complete state of misery for what seemed like forever. I held Zachary in my arms and sat there, staring at my floor-length mirror in anger at my misshapen, postpartum, overweight body, crying about my life.

I wondered how on earth I got here. I was tired, sad, lonely, frustrated, angry, and every emotion you can name. I felt an overwhelming sense of guilt about how I had treated my children, and I was beating myself up for my childish behavior.

We moms sure know how to kick ourselves when we're down, and that's exactly what I did. If I could tell this overwhelmed mom something now, I would grab her by the shoulders, look her straight in the eyes, and say, "Stop being so hard on yourself, woman! This is the hardest job ever, and you're doing the best you can, and that's enough."

Sitting there, I was so aware that I wanted out, but I didn't know what that even meant. Not that I was suicidal or even depressed, although I do fully understand how some moms can get to that place, and I completely empathize with them. Having kids is a shocking change and far from easy.

It was more that I wanted relief from the exhaustion and deep sadness that came with the daily grind of diapers and cleaning and feeding and not sleeping and coffee and more coffee and being alone and tired with fussy kids all the time.

I wondered, *Is this what life with kids will be like for me forever? Is there not more to my life?* I had a career I wanted to get back to, and I felt stuck. I also felt so extremely self conscious in my post-baby body. I was overweight and far too impatient with the weight loss process. I worried I may be stuck in an uncomfortable body and life forever.

I knew I needed something, but I had no idea what that something even was. I entertained the thoughts of regretting having children if this was what having children was like. I then felt even more guilt for having such horrible thoughts. However, it wasn't them; it was me. I had this mom thing all wrong. I just didn't know it yet.

As I sat there crying, I missed the freedom that came with my old kid-free life. I missed my fit, lean body and fitting into my old clothes, and above all, feeling good in my skin. I missed being able to exercise. I missed conversing with adults. I missed having time for myself. I missed sleep. I missed feeling happy. I missed my friends and my freedom. I missed feeling like myself. Where did she go? I felt so lost and out of touch with who I even was anymore. I had become Mom but neglected Alison.

Somehow, every emotion and situation in my life culminated, and on that day, at that moment, I was done with living my life this way. I was done, and yet, I rationally knew I could never be done, so I felt trapped, suffocated, isolated, and frustrated all at once. I was so overwhelmed by the weight of caring for three kids and not caring for myself.

Hearing my kids announce, "Dad is home," gave me instant peace. I could hear the immediate calm in Andrew and Levi's voice. It felt as if a weight had just been lifted off all of our shoulders.

When Graham knocked at the bathroom door, I thanked God I didn't have to do this alone. I opened the door and quickly handed him the baby. I continued to cry uncontrollably despite feeling some relief by his presence. When we made eye contact, he asked me what I needed, and more tears came flooding down. Though I didn't know the answer, the question itself made me feel totally supported and loved, and I certainly needed both at that moment.

That very question would be pivotal in my coming out of the dark place I had fallen into. He stayed to hug me and then took the kids and left me alone where I wanted to be. As I sat on the bathroom floor kid free, crying like a child, I was overwhelmed by that question. Overwhelmed and terrified because I could not find the answer.

How could I not even know what I needed? How could I be that out of touch with myself? I knew I needed sleep, a kid free shower, an adult conversation, and a day without bickering children, but I didn't know what I needed to become happy again, to feel good again, to feel like my old self again. I was so disconnected with what I needed to get back to myself. The old me felt so far away. I felt lost.

Climbing out of that dark place took time and work and a lot of Graham's help and support. It was far from an overnight change. I do not even know where I would be without him in my corner. I'm certain God knew I would need Graham. His help was life changing. He is skilled in a lot of areas and mindset coaching is one of them. I can imagine he never expected needing to work with his wife when he studied at university, but I am so thankful he had these skills. His help, along with a lot of prayers, love, support, exercise, healthy eating and having my needs met, helped me find my way back home.

I asked myself these questions daily. *What do I need today to feel good? What do I need to feel rested, calm, and happy? What do I need to ensure I am healthy for everyone who needs me? Am I getting what I need? Are my needs being prioritized the way I prioritize my children and everyone and everything else?*

I had been running around like a chicken with my head cut off, looking after everyone else's needs without having ever met my own. I was trying to hold so many things up, but I had forgotten that I needed to be included in the pile. In fact, I was the foundation of that pile.

Neglecting myself eventually led to this crash. Sometimes, it takes crashing to realize something isn't working. I had no idea things needed to be fixed until I was broken on my bathroom floor.

In hindsight, this moment would be used to help so many other moms come out of their dark places and find themselves again. So, I am thankful for it. Because it happened, I could reach my hand back and help others lighten their loads and enjoy being moms rather than suffering through it.

At the time, though, this was one of the most challenging moments of my life. The realization I had in that moment and the days and weeks and years that followed was that it was time for me to stop living the lie that a good mom gives herself away and, instead, believe that a good mom looks after herself, too. I needed to become a healthy mom who puts her needs first and then meets the needs of her children. Once I did this, so much changed.

There was a calm deep inside my soul that swept through our entire home. I yelled less often. I cried a lot less, and I was happy and excited about being a mom for the first time in much too long. I was more patient. I was more grateful. I got healthier both mentally and physically. I lost the fifty-five pounds I had gained from my third pregnancy. I had more energy, and above all, I felt like myself again. The me I had lost when I became a mom and forgot about Alison.

It wasn't long after things in my home got better that Graham and I both agreed we needed to share this story with moms. We both had this overwhelming sense of urgency to help moms everywhere learn how to care for themselves and not feel guilty about it.

Children deserve to have the very best of their mom, and moms deserve to be their very best. We both knew that we could be a part of helping that happen for moms.

So, we began *The Switch Project*, an online fitness, food, and lifestyle program that helps moms switch from last to first on their priority list. We've since helped countless moms become healthier and happier and learn that it is not selfish to take care of themselves, too. It's necessary.

Moms are the most important people to their children. They can influence so many lives and impact the world in a major way, but first, they need to be liberated, loved, and have their needs met.

It would be easy to say the story ends there. It sounds like a happy ending, right? But this is where the story begins. Because of my crash, I was given this beautiful gift of awareness of all the things I had been carrying. I had no clue that worrying was one of them, but I was finally open enough to evaluate how I had been choosing to live. I was at a new place where I was ready to take a hard look at everything that I had been carrying. This openness was the key to the awareness that changed my life.

The years that have followed this pivotal moment for me have been soul-searching years. They have been eye opening, healing, and filled with incredible lessons, and I know I am now at a place I can share from. Once we've survived the storm, we can see so much clearer, and from a better vantage point, we can help others through their storms.

Despite setting down the obligation to cater to everyone else's needs and setting down the notion that caring for myself first is selfish, there was something I hadn't set down yet, and it was only because I didn't even know I was holding it. There are so many things we carry with no awareness. Often, they are the heaviest and most exhausting.

Despite discovering more peace, learning to make myself a priority, and helping other moms do the same, I still hadn't set down the habit of worry, and it was stealing from my kids and me in a major way.

I needed to stop worrying so much about what could go wrong and start focussing on all the things that are going right, right now. But first, I needed to realize that this was a habit I had picked up and allowed to become a part of me.

Some days, I am so far away from worrying that I even forget it is something I struggled with. Some days, I slip back into old ways, and the familiarity haunts me. Every day, I'm relieved that I am aware enough and, therefore, far enough away from it, so I can choose to step off the worry wheel before I get spinning too far in the wrong direction. In doing so, I am also choosing not to pass this destructive pattern on to my children. I'm thankful to be closer to the healthy side of this life-stealing, joy-sucking, habit.

Sometimes, we don't even realize just how free we are until we're faced with the chance to look back and see how far we've come. This opportunity came recently when we were looking at purchasing our dream home in the country. We were quickly outgrowing our tiny bungalow and its little backyard, and I had always lived with this dream to have some property in the country with trees and space for my three boys to run free in.

After a miraculous chain of events and some divine timing, I found the home, and my husband and I made an offer. As we waited to hear if it had been accepted, I shared my excitement about discovering our dream home with my dad.

As I did, I was more aware than ever just how far away I was from worry, and how much he was in it but didn't even know.

When we've been set free, we can see so much clearer what we were victims of. We can also recognize it in others more than we ever could before. I think this is such a gift because it allows us the opportunity to help them find their way out, too.

I believe our struggles are not just for ourselves. The lessons we gain can help those around us who may struggle with similar challenges. When we have been liberated, we can see so much clearer. And the wisdom we've acquired through our challenges allows us to reach our hand back and help others through theirs, if they'll let us help.

I told my father about how the country home has so many trees and so much space and a wonderful fifteen-foot pond. I explained it is a corner lot just off a highway and has a wood-burning fireplace, which Graham was most excited about. I went on and on because the excitement was overflowing, and then I ran into his caution sign, which could have easily become my stop sign had I let it.

His voice interrupted my enthusiasm like a hammer. "Wait a minute," he said. "All that sounds great, but what about that pond and fireplace and highway?" My dad wasn't so quick to jump into my excitement parade.

Instead, he was worried one of my kids could drown in the pond and shared this concern with me. He also expressed his feelings about the wood-burning fireplace and the potential danger of the location just off of a highway. I know he was simply being a caring father who was cautiously supportive. Though I know they came from a place of love, his questions felt more like punches to me. When you worry about so much so often, and others express their worries, you can easily take them on yourself, and that's exactly what I was fighting the urge to do.

"What if that fireplace is a fire hazard? Can the boys swim well yet? Do you have lifejackets for them, and have they completed water safety training? How close is the highway? Are they biking on it? Do they know to stay away from it?"

Though they were, and are, absolutely valid and reasonable concerns, they could easily become my fears if I let them. It doesn't take much to let them snowball into sleepless nights and obsessive helicopter-mom tendencies, if I'm not mindful. I could feel the pull to fear all the what ifs.

There's a reason the Bible commands us to, "cast down every high thing that exalts itself against the knowledge of God, bringing every thought into captivity to the obedience of Christ." (2 Corinthians 10:5) God knew we would face these kinds of challenges, and He wanted us to be equipped and ready to combat them with his truths rather than suffer in fear under lies.

As soon as my dad spoke these what if's, the temptation to leap into worry was so powerful. Fear is tangible and contagious. For a few moments, I let my mind drift to horror scenes of my children getting hit by a car or drowning or screaming because of a fire, but then I stopped myself and interrupted the irrational thoughts. I grabbed them and said out loud, "No way! I refuse to go there."

My husband walked into our kitchen to the sound of me affirming, "I will not live my life in fear. I will not hold my children back worrying about what could go wrong. I will not stop living because I'm afraid of what could happen if I do."

"Good." He responded and then carried on his way with an understanding smile for my need to make this verbal declaration to gain control of my thoughts. This is one tool in my toolbox that has helped me, and regardless of how I look to others, I sometimes need to confront the thoughts out loud. Our brains listen when we speak. Worries can't be present when we override them with rational declarations. Sometimes, it's important to stop fear in its tracks with our very own voice. God gave us the power to override every thought.

My dad's concerns were valid and wise, but I had to choose not to let them take away my sleep or my excitement for our dream home. We went over fire safety with our kids and made sure we had our smoke and carbon monoxide alarms up to date. I purchased a lifesaver ring for our pond, life jackets for each child, and booked swimming lessons. I also taught my children safety about the pond and the highway. That is the extent to it all. That's where I will set it down and let it go. I refuse to let it rob me.

I can't live my life in peace and joy if I sit in my home and keep my kids at my side worried that if I let them play and run free and be curious and explore, something bad could happen. I refuse to live that way any longer. I've wasted too many years like that already, and I won't lose one more day.

I can educate them, and then I can move on and let them be free to be kids and trust they are in God's hands. Otherwise, my fears and worries will quickly become theirs, and that's not fair to them.

The worrying habit stops with me, and for the first time in several years, I can see that it actually has stopped. Years ago, I may have not even purchased the house because my fears would have prevented me from being free to have faith that we will all be safe.

The good news is that the offer for our dream home was accepted, and rather than worry, I celebrated. Moving to this house has been one of the best decisions in my entire life. I am so grateful for it and am so happy I didn't let worry keep me or my family from it. Sometimes, we miss out on incredible opportunities because we let what if stand in our way. We can miss out on what could be over a fear of what may never happen.

Our new home is surrounded by beautiful country roads lined with tall trees. I love running and recently went for a scenic and memorable country run. It's something I enjoy doing a few times a week to stay healthy and clear my mind; this is another great tool in my toolbox.

On this day, I was feeling extra energized, so I did the full country block, rather than the short out and back I usually do. As I was approaching the corner that was the homestretch, I recalled another country run I had done many years earlier before I had children. It was one I can never forget because I had come one millimetre away from an emergency air lift and possible death.

It happened when I was in my early twenties. I set out to fulfill my dream of running a marathon and was more than ready. I had done several half marathons and felt prepared to make the leap to the full forty-two-kilometre distance.

To train for the marathon, I ran on country roads. I liked the scenery and the lack of traffic. On this day, I was planning to do an out and back for a total of thirty kilometres. I was ten kilometres in and having the time of my life. My music was cranked, and I was singing along with it—probably off key but with no care in the world. I was feeling fantastic and was on track for a personal best time. I felt fast and free.

I had no idea what was about to happen. I didn't get a bad feeling in the pit of my stomach. I didn't have a feeling come over me that I should turn around. There was no forewarning, so I ran in happy oblivion, completely unaware of the attack that was just up ahead.

The highway wasn't busy, but to be safe, I ran close to the side of the road. Perhaps a little too close. I remember the sound of a loud growl interrupting my music, and with no time to react, I remember looking down in absolute shock as a giant black dog's jaw clenched onto the side of my leg. I remember screaming at the top of my lungs, and then I remember feeling something pour down the side of my leg as I tried hard to shake this massive dog off me.

Oddly enough, I didn't feel pain at all. Maybe that was a God thing, or maybe I was in total shock. Either way, I distinctly remember awaiting the pain to hit me, but it didn't. At the sound of my screams, a man came out of his farmhouse and called the dog off me. I told him what had happened, and his response was not at all what I expected it to be.

He said, "You're fine; it's just a little scratch." Shaking uncontrollably, I rolled up my black and pink tights to see what the dog had done to me and looked in horror. I could see the inside of my leg. There was an extremely deep, two-inch gaping wound. It wasn't just a little scratch; I needed medical attention.

I explained I had to go to the hospital, and he tried to convince me I was making a bigger deal out of things than I needed to. As I told him his dog could get put down for this, he shared with me that the dog had attacked a child the week before, and he was sorry he didn't have it on a leash.

I was angry. I tried to focus my energy on calling my husband instead of yelling at the man. Once I knew Graham was on his way, I looked back to tell the man that I was going to have to report his dog, and that's when his granddaughter came out of the house and limped toward me. As she got closer, I could see that she only had one leg; the other was a prosthetic. She had tears in her eyes and pleaded with me, "He's my best friend. Please don't put my best friend down."

I told her that her best friend can't attack people, and she agreed with that. My heart was torn. I was angry and sad and obviously didn't want this child to lose her dog. No doubt she had already been through something traumatic. I didn't want to add to it.

She grabbed my hand and begged me to save her best friend. I could see tears in her eyes, and I felt her desperation for her dog. She loved him. Suddenly, the pain set in. I took my hand and applied pressure to the wound.

Graham pulled up, wrote the address down, and took me to the hospital. As the doctor inspected the wound, he paused for a second and looked me in the eye and said, "Wow." Then he explained, "The dogs tooth missed your joint capsule and femoral artery by literally a hair. You're so lucky. You could have bled out on the side of the road."

The good news is that I was okay. Glue sealed the wound shut, antibiotics took care of any chance of infection, and my recovery was quick. I was set back only a few weeks and could continue my training and complete the marathon.

As for the dog, the hospital reported it and had it quarantined for two weeks. They ended up keeping him alive but with the rule that he needed to be on a leash at all times.

I was terrified to run in the country, and by terrified, I mean I finished all my training indoors on a treadmill. That's what fear can do. It can keep us indoors forever if we let it.

As I did my recent country run near our new home, I was reflecting on this scary event, and literally minutes later, I heard a barking dog. I looked up to see it crossing the highway on its way toward me, and it didn't look friendly. It growled.

For a second, I was terrified, but then I stopped my fear and yelled at the top of my lungs, "No! Go home!" I was shocked to witness the dog abruptly stop at the middle line and turn around and do exactly what I told him to do. Thankfully!

Though I may run with some sort of bear spray from this point forward, I refuse to stop running on country roads. I refuse to let the fear and worry of what could happen keep me from enjoying life.

If our children fall off their bikes and scrape their knees, we encourage them to be brave, get back on, and try again. In fact, we wouldn't let them decide based on a few scraped knees to never ride a bike again. We wouldn't let them get away with allowing their fear to steal the joy their bikes bring them. Yet, as adults, we often let the fall keep us down. The fall prevents us from getting back up and trying again. In fact, the fall gives us a valid reason to never try again at all.

We can't live our life afraid of falling. If we do, we'll miss out on flying. There is so much to gain when we choose to get back up. With every country run, I am taking back what worry and fear could have stolen from me. I am making the choice to not allow worry to keep me on a treadmill or, worse, prevent me from ever doing another run again.

As you can see, I have come so far. The good news is that you can come with me. There is so much more living to do on the other side of fear. "For God has not given us a spirit of fear but of power and of love and of a sound mind." (2 Timothy 1:7)

He wants us to be wise and make good choices and take control over our minds, but he doesn't want us to be gripped by the fist of worry. You'll miss out on the best days if you spend them worrying about the worst ones.

So, my questions to you are simple; what country roads are you avoiding because you're afraid of a dog? What amazing opportunities could you be blocking in your life because you're too worried about what could go wrong? What could you be preventing your children from experiencing for the same reason?

Without awareness, we simply cannot break any habit we have. You probably know someone who does something repetitively, and they aren't even aware they do it. Maybe that someone is you. Maybe, like me, you've been worrying, and you weren't even fully aware of just how much.

There are so many things we carry around. They are heavy, but we don't notice how heavy until we set them down. I hope that my liberation isn't just for me and my children. Read on and allow yourself to reflect, be open, learn, and examine your thoughts and habits, and my liberation can also be yours. Freedom can flow if we let it.

Life is much too short to let what ifs keep you from living it. *What is* is the only thing that matters, and if we worry, we will not only block all the amazing things that could be, but we will also miss out on all that is right now. It's time to break the habit.

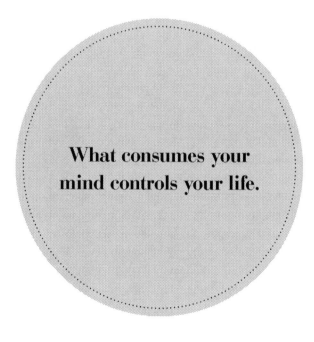

What consumes your
mind controls your life.

CHAPTER 2

Fire

Worry is like a fire. The more we feed it, the more it grows. The more it grows, the more powerful it becomes, and if left unattended, it can easily overtake everything around it. Eventually, what we could once control, we no longer can.

Fire consumes. So does worry. If we're not careful, it will steal inches. First our thoughts, then our sleep, then it will inch toward our peace, and over time, it will consume our joy and entire life. We will stop living our life to its fullest without even knowing it. We'll miss out on what is and what could be all because of what if. This is what happened to me.

I once witnessed a plane crash. Before we had kids, Graham and I lived at a lake. He was walking our dog while I was cleaning our kitchen. We were both startled by a sudden thunderous sound directly above us. It was so loud and sudden that I dropped the broom and ran outside to see what it was.

I watched as thick black smoke trailed across the sky behind a tiny plane heading straight for the middle of the lake. The engine was loud and sounded like it was ripping the sky open.

Seconds later, we both witnessed the plane smash into the water, with an echo I'll never forget, and break in half when it hit. Then I heard a man screaming for help. I held my breath as

I watched what can only be described as a horror movie play out in front of me.

It was late autumn, and it was freezing outside. All the boats were in storage for the winter. No one could help the man screaming for help.

The water was ice cold, and we watched in shock from the edge of our dock as the plane sank into it and take this stranger with it. A desperate voice pierced the silence again, yelling, "Help me! Please, someone help me," but no one could get to him in time. In a matter of seconds, he disappeared, leaving behind a chilling emptiness and the sound of his screams on replay in my head.

I've never felt so helpless. We called 911, knowing it was too late. We watched as neighbors across the lake scrambled to unpack their canoes too late. We stood frozen at the edge of our dock, begging for someone to do something, but we all knew that no one could. He was too far away, and there was nothing that any of us could have done to save him.

I found out later that he was a firefighter in his late seventies who lived a long and fulfilled life with children and a loving wife. He died doing what he loved to do. It broke my heart that he had spent years helping others, and when he needed help the most, no one came to answer his call, but I justified it all with knowing that he was old and loved.

I thought knowing he lived a long and happy life and died doing what he loved to do would make it all easier for me to get over it. I thought it would be the consolation that I needed to move on from the trauma I had witnessed. But then I let worry keep me from living.

I didn't go to California with my husband on his business trip. Then I didn't go to Mexico with him for a one-week vacation at a beautiful resort. Then I didn't go to Peru and climb Machu Picchu—all because of what if?

Life is meant to be lived, but when we let our thoughts about what could happen rule it, we slowly allow our life to be set on a safe, risk-free shelf, and don't even realize that in doing so, we miss out on all the amazing opportunities it has to offer.

I told myself excellent stories about why I didn't go on the trips with my husband, and I believed them. *I was busy raising kids. Someone needed to stay home with the baby. Someone needed to run the business. I'll go next time.* Fear can sound very practical and give us rational reasons we shouldn't do something, and that's exactly what it did.

Every trip Graham took brought me sleepless nights. Add the horrendous events of 911 to this traumatic plane crash and you can imagine where my mind would venture to. While he was flying, I was worrying myself into an absolute state of exhaustion and throwing more logs on the fire with every thought I had.

Because I started believing my worries were real, I sent him messages mid-flight to make sure I had said proper goodbyes. Worry can take what if and make it feel so real that your mind starts to believe your fears are going to happen. It's incredible how convincing it can be.

Once I knew his flight had landed safely, the worrying would stop for a little while. At least until the next flight. I was stuck in a cycle. I didn't consciously know I had a fear of flying or that I suffered from posttraumatic stress disorder. I wasn't fully aware of how much I worried, either. I discovered all this many years later when I wanted to visit a friend who was a two-hour flight away from me.

In a moment of bravery, I booked the tickets, and then the bravery faded and the cycle began again. The weeks and days leading up to the flight, I fought hard to sleep while the worry reel played awful movies in my head. I feared the plane crashing and allowed myself to entertain the horror of never seeing my kids again. The detail my mind made up was horrific. The imagination, if left to its own wandering, can paint pictures so real you can feel them in your body. That's what mine did.

What if the pilot has a heart attack or is a terrorist? What if the plane gets struck by lightning? The endless loop robbed my sleep as I allowed irrational questions to invade my head.

As if that wasn't bad enough, I even Googled how fast a plane travels so I could evaluate the likelihood of surviving a crash. (Never Google how fast a plane flies if you're worried about flying. It will definitely not calm you down.)

I never shared this struggle with Graham, although he knew I was terrified of flying. In hindsight, I should have at least prayed about it. It wasn't a secret to God. Obviously, He already knew my struggles, but rather than share them and pray for help, I let them fester and grow and consume my peace and sleep.

I knew they sounded irrational when I said them out loud. I knew they were impractical and far fetched. I knew they weren't a normal experience to be having. So, to not look like I was some kind of lunatic, I kept them well hidden and put on an excellent front.

Why do we smile over sadness? Flex through weakness? Hide our struggles? And tell our loved ones we're fine when we aren't? Maybe we care more about what others will think than we care for ourselves and our wellbeing. Or maybe we feel like we don't want to add to anyone else's already full pile. I'm uncertain which, but I know this; I did a fantastic job of faking bravery, that is, until the actual flight time arrived.

I forced myself on that plane because my desire to see my friend and be there for her during a challenging post-partum time was greater than my desire to avoid planes. It was there on that plane as I took my seat and waited for take-off that I had my first ever panic attack and my prayers answered, in that exact order.

The plane took off, and we immediately headed into some turbulence, which certainly helped initiate the panic. My palms got sweaty, my heart raced, my mind raced faster than my heart, and I breathed heavily. It felt like I couldn't quite get a full breath. With every bounce and jolt the plane made, I became more tense and lightheaded.

I placed my seat back and pretended to relax so the people around me wouldn't wonder what was wrong. On the outside, I may have appeared calm, but inside, I was panicking. I tried to count backward from ten and focus on slowing my breathing down. I was already out of control of my thoughts, and now, for the first time, I also felt out of control of my body.

Then, ironically or not, a woman's voice interrupted my panic with words I'll never forget: "Your fear of flying is a fear of being out of control. The sooner you realize you're in control of very little, the more peace you'll have in your life. I'm a psychologist, and I can tell you from experience, trying to be in control will cage you forever. It's letting go that will set you free." I was shocked and somehow forced out a thanks.

Have you ever heard God's voice so loud and clear it totally snapped you out of whatever you were in? That was this moment for me. I can't fully explain it, but I felt her words go into my soul. I know this was a God moment. In this case, He was speaking through this wonderful woman who never said another word to me on the flight. Instead, she slept peacefully. But she didn't need to say another word. Enough was said. The message was received loud and clear.

My panic melted away as I prayed, "God, thank you for knowing just what I needed to hear. Please help me end this fear of flying and constant worrying and to rest knowing you are in control, and I am not. Help me let go."

When the truth speaks, we know it's the truth, and if we are willing to embrace it, it can set us free. In that moment, I realized I had let my worry about planes burn up all the joy that could be experienced from seeing the world. I had been letting worry prevent me from living. Just as she had spoken, my desire to be in control needed to be set aside.

This whole time, I had made excuses why I couldn't fly because I was afraid to do it. It took facing that fear to realize how bad it really was. Sometimes, we must do the very thing we're terrified to do to fully overcome it. Sometimes, we must learn that what we are worrying about won't happen.

Facing the fear also meant facing the regret of missed opportunities and the willingness to be brave and face new ones. As I jumped around on that turbulent flight, the memory of the crash came rushing back to me. I thought about how out of control the man on the plane was as he faced his last breath. I allowed myself to experience all the emotions the memory brought with it, and then I let it all go.

As I did, I was so aware of how out of control I had let my worrying get. I realized all that matters is who is in control, and I believe that is God. I also believe He uses people to speak to us and help us overcome our internal struggles, and on that flight, He did exactly that.

Much like a sudden rush of adrenaline, I felt a brand-new sense of calm come over my entire body. I can't explain it; I just felt different. It was a sense of peace I had only ever experienced once before. I got off of that flight with so much more awareness about my worrying habit and with a newfound calm. One that I had longed for many years to have. I can only explain it as a gift from God because it didn't go away. I believe my prayer was answered, and I was free from so much of the fear that had gripped me for so many years.

I can never get the trips that I missed back, but the next year, I vacationed with my husband in Mexico for the first time in almost nine years. Then I visited my parents in South Carolina and attended a business conference in Las Vegas. All three trips were amazing. Each time, I realized I had been missing out on so much fun and adventure by letting worry dictate my decisions. I'll never get back the years I avoided flying, but I'm so thankful to have the future back.

This wasn't a magical fix. Plane rides haven't been easy, but they've definitely been better, and that counts. I practice gratitude during the takeoff. I say a prayer. I sit back and focus on all the great things I'll do when I get home, and I trust God has me in his hands, exactly where I belong.

And guess what? It works. One time, I even fell asleep on the plane in the middle of the day. My mind can still wander if I let it, but when it does, I feel much more in control because I know who has me, and I have a new awareness that I never had before. One I believe I got from facing my fear head on and letting God speak into my situation.

I'm so thankful for all the memories and life I have gained from having stepped past worry to decide not to let it steal from me any longer. I'm also thankful for a God who knew what I needed when I needed it. He truly answers our prayers.

Worry, like fire, must be actively put out. We must consciously decide that we are done with living our life this way. It will require action and effort, but it can happen. The fire we feed is the one that will grow, and the fire we put out is the one that will die. Much like a fire, it may not die right away. It will still smoulder and flicker, and the coal and ashes will take time to lose their heat, their power over you. However, eventually, the more you starve that fire of worry, the less you will worry.

If we let worry blaze, it will consume so much of our lives to the extent that we will stop living them entirely. We will make choices based on worry. We will eventually build so many what-if walls around ourselves that we will be trapped in a safe, risk-free prison cell we mistake for living.

This almost happened to Samantha Bloom. I recently watched the movie about her called *Penguin Bloom*. It's a true story about a competitive surfer named Samantha, who went on a vacation with her family and fell off a roof-top patio. She broke her back and became paralyzed from the chest down.

To help her overcome the intense mental struggle of not being able to compete as a surfer anymore and to help her come to terms with life in a wheelchair, her husband hired a canoe coach for her.

Her mom was worried. Samantha obviously couldn't swim

like she used to, and her mom expressed her fear about the canoe tipping and her possibly drowning. What she didn't understand was that her daughter was already drowning. The lifeline was the canoe coach. Her husband knew it. He spoke up from his soul and said something we all need to consider, saying, "We don't live in what if. We *live* our lives." His words were powerful and cut through her mother's fears.

Samantha became a national canoe sprint champion and is now also a world champion surfer. She went from drowning in the prison of her circumstances to being an amazing athlete. Had she never gotten into the canoe, she would have never achieved such great feats.

She is an inspiration to so many people, and we can all take many lessons from her incredible story. The one that stands out most to me is this: Don't let your fear of drowning keep you from getting in the water. Maybe the fear of drowning is actually drowning you, and the water is the life line needed to live free from fear.

We have the power to take our lives back. The choice is absolutely ours to make. We can choose to allow worries to steal the living we were meant to do and hold us back from all the amazing experiences life offers us, or we can choose to live life instead.

The good news is that if worry is your battlefield, awareness is your weapon. When you can realize what you are afraid of, you can do something I just recently discovered; you can evaluate the validity and probability of your fears actually happening.

I recently heard Pastor Holly Furtick talk about how her mom taught her to rationalize her fears. She shared how she lived in Florida, and it was common to have big storms there. She remembered when she was little being afraid of the storms, but she also remembered her mom never seemed afraid. She expressed how she was thankful that her mom taught her how to rationalize her fears.

I never even knew this was something we could teach our children until I heard her say it. Something clicked for me when she spoke. When we have the awareness of our worries and fears, we can then take the time to rationalize them, weigh their probability, and navigate through the faulty logic they are founded upon.

It's like turning the light on for a child sitting afraid in the dark. Suddenly, shadows and shapes that appeared scary in the dark make sense in the light. Fears and worries that once appeared big become smaller and even seem silly when we can see them for what they are—lies.

Imagine being able to teach your children to do this too. How freeing it would be to be able to stop in the middle of a what-if tantrum and bring solid wisdom into the conversation. This is what I realized we can do. Listing out every worry you have and then taking the time to read it aloud and rationalize it is yet another tool in the toolbox to overcome worry. Think about the probability, and you'll worry less.

Certainly, some concerns are valid, but even so, it doesn't mean they are factual. Our minds have the capability to trail off on a tangent if we allow them to do so, but we have power over our minds. What we focus on is what we will see more of and is what will grow. The more you feed the fire of peace, the more peace you will have.

Moms do so much for so many people. They give so much love and joy and time to their children; they need the calm that comes with letting worry go. Letting go frees up space for living. Putting out this blaze of worry isn't easy, and there's not a one size fits all approach, but I want to share what has worked for me in hopes that it could also work for you.

Instead of feeding worry, I've now chosen a different fire, one that brings me joy and peace and a deep sense of calm. It's how I've slowly put the other one out. It's an acronym and goes like this.

F is for faith, which is my foundation and the only reason I can live worry free.

I is for inner work, which we all need to do.

R is for real food, which helps keep our bodies and minds clear and healthy.

E is for exercise, which ensures our bodies and minds stay strong, healthy, and stress free.

Not only am I feeding this new fire, but I'm also walking around with a pack of matches in my hand so I can strike a few for every worrying mom who crosses my path. The more I talk about it with fellow moms, the more I realize worrying and moms go together like toddlers and sticky fingers. It's common, more common than I ever realized.

I will elaborate in the coming pages and share with you this new fire I've learned to feed. It's the one that grows bigger in my life every day, and it will absolutely help you step through the fire you've allowed to get out of hand in your life and kindle a new, much healthier one.

Here's the deal; I'll strike the match for you, but it's up to you to keep the fire going. That requires a choice to stop letting worry dictate how you live your life and start actually living it instead.

I can't guarantee you'll make this choice once, and it'll be smooth sailing after that. However, I can absolutely guarantee that making this choice will be a start, and like anything, you don't have to be great to start, but you have to start to be great. I hope that this is your start to living worry free. Old habits die hard, but they can and will die when you starve them and feed new, healthier ones instead.

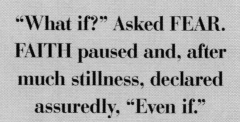

"What if?" Asked FEAR.
FAITH paused and, after
much stillness, declared
assuredly, "Even if."

Faith

Are you leaning on faith or giving in to fear? Are you trusting in God, or are you trusting your worries instead? Is your assurance in hope or hopelessness? There really isn't much room for grey. We either veer to one side or the other. Oxford Languages Dictionary defines faith as "complete trust or confidence in someone or something." Complete, meaning absolutely all of your trust.

Where are you placing your confidence? Sometimes, we place more faith in the storm surrounding us than we do in the one who has the power to calm it. One can be seen with our natural eyes, and the other requires a belief in things unseen. One perpetuates fear, and the other brings a peace that surpasses all understanding. Both are a choice we make even if we don't realize it.

Adrian Rogers so profoundly said, "Worry looks at God through the circumstances. Peace looks at circumstances through God." Too often, I have chosen to worry over choosing to have faith that regardless of the circumstances, God has me in his hands.

There are countless nights I should have just gone to sleep instead of wasting my time and energy trying to control the outcome by attempting to explore and analyze every worst-case scenario. Trust me on this, I am still very much a work in progress. Perfection often feels so far away.

More often than not, my imagination conjured up far worse circumstances than I was actually in. The story I'm about to share is no exception. I absolutely imagined it to be catastrophically worse than it ever got. This doesn't negate that it was bad, but in hindsight, I wish I would have chosen to trust God and have peace instead of giving in to the temptation to worry. I'm sharing my struggle in hopes it will ignite your faith.

I was seven months pregnant with our third son when my husband and I got a phone call that shattered our world as we knew it. It was one of those life moments where we knew right away that nothing would ever be the same again.

At the time, we were operating the fitness and wellness centre my mom had started. We had taken on running it for just over nine years. I had worked in it off and on for sixteen years, starting as a front desk attendant when I was in high school and then as a personal trainer throughout university. It was a huge part of my life and, in so many ways, changed my life for the better.

It began after my mom left her nursing career. She moved ahead in faith with a vision for a preventative health centre. She wanted to help people live healthier, and so did I. I absolutely loved being a part of it in every way.

Graham and I had worked in it through a massive expansion from a tiny gym to a ten-thousand-square-foot fully equipped facility with a large team and member base. Fitness was, and is, our passion, and we absolutely loved what we got to do there. I couldn't imagine my life without it but was soon about to.

The phone rang, interrupting what had been a relaxing Friday. I had my feet up watching our two young boys building towers with Legos just minutes before their bedtime. Graham answered the phone, and I knew something was wrong right away.

He tried to be subtle. He slowly moved into the other room where I could still see him, but he quieted his voice so I wouldn't hear the conversation. His tone was very serious, and as he distanced himself physically, I leaned in to catch whatever snippet of the conversation I could. I knew something wasn't right.

I've heard the expression that colour can drain from someone's face, but this was the first time I witnessed it happen in real time. While he listened on the phone, I watched out of the corner of my eye as my husband's usual pink cheeks turned white. His happy demeanor and calm smile were suddenly replaced with a confused, blank stare and a tense grip on the phone.

I waited impatiently to find out what was going on and was relieved to see him finally hang up. I knew he was trying hard to protect me from the blow he had just received. I had been having some early labor challenges and was told to reduce my stress load so the baby would stay put for a few more months.

I knew there was no way that he could shelter me from whatever had just smacked him in the face. It was much too obvious and too late for him to try to hide it. Rather than explain, he said, "It's going to be okay." His body language, pale face, and tone of voice told me otherwise. I didn't believe him, and in fact, I believed the opposite.

His response only left me more concerned. "What is?!" I begged for the information. Before he could speak, I quickly jumped to, "Who died?" It had suddenly hit me that my entire family was on a cruise, so of course my worrying mind raced to thinking the boat had sunk.

Jumping from a phone conversation to the death of my entire family happened in mere seconds, and if I didn't get answers soon, I was likely about to be planning funerals and asking how I will ever manage life with no family left. He could see me getting worked up, so he tried forcing the words out but could barely get them off his tongue. "The gym. We are out."

I was so confused. Naturally, I asked him to explain, but he was speechless. He walked into the living room and sat down so fast it looked as if his legs gave out from under him. In hindsight, I think they actually did. The couch cushioned his collapse into it, and I watched as he placed his head into his hands. He was motionless and white. He looked like a statue sitting in our living room.

After what felt like hours, but was more like minutes, he was able to choke the words out and explain what had happened. In a series of heartbreaking events, the gym we had worked so hard to grow was gone.

Just like that, in the blink of an eye, we had both lost our income, our investments, and the business we had been working so hard to build. It was sold to a third party, and we were left at seven-months pregnant, with two kids to feed, a baby soon to arrive, a new home to pay for, a private school to fund, and zero family income.

With no notice or severance, we lost everything we had poured so many years into building. This included so many wonderful people who we loved wholeheartedly. It was a second home to us, and we gave it our energy, passion, time, and love. We never even got to say goodbye.

We were not in a place financially or emotionally to tackle legal claims, and I didn't have the heart for that, anyway. This was just a hit we would have to figure out how to take; one we hadn't seen coming and did not know how we would ever navigate through.

I sat down beside Graham to absorb the blow with him. My very pregnant body already felt heavy, but now it felt as if someone had placed bricks on top of my chest. I couldn't get a full breath, and I was in absolute shock.

As I watched my two small boys innocently play together on the carpet, completely unaware of what had just happened, fear flooded my thoughts. I felt the third baby boy jump around in my belly, and the irrational, unrelenting worry began.

Immediately, I was hit with the massive weight of what if. *What if we lose absolutely everything and wind up homeless with three kids?* My mind sprinted past the practical thought that things would be tight for a little while, but we would get through this and right toward home foreclosures, car repossessions, and not being able to feed my children.

As it turns out, there's a whole new dimension to worry, a level I had never been worried enough to meet until now. This worry wasn't the same as having a human in my belly. It was literally paralyzing. It robbed my appetite, took away my sleep, and stole my joy. Couple that with a completely broken heart, and to say I was in rough shape would be a massive understatement.

The more I worried, the less I could breathe. My heart raced, my entire body sweat, and then, at seven months pregnant, I started experiencing painful contractions, ones I knew weren't Braxton Hicks. This unexpected explosion in the middle of our life definitely put me over the edge physically and emotionally.

Worry is powerful. We think it's just in our heads, but it transfers immediately into our bodies, too. We physically carry it, and it has a tangible impact. It affects our mood, our blood pressure, our lung capacity, our muscles, our ability to think straight, and, in my case, my unborn child.

I regret the contractions didn't wake me up enough to make me realize I needed to calm down. The truth is, though, I couldn't calm down. I was completely out of control. I didn't have the tools I have now, and I lacked any awareness that I was even doing it. When life got rocky, I worried.

So, rather than calming down, I did the opposite and slid entirely out of control of my thoughts and emotions. I let my default setting take over completely and worried myself into an absolute state of anxiety.

It's a slippery slope. Worry leads to panic fairly quickly. With the onset of contractions came even more worry. *What if I have this baby too early? What if we lose our home, and I have a premature child that I can't even afford to care for? What if the baby doesn't even make it through this night? What if I don't either?*

Fear gripped me, and as all the worst-case scenarios snowballed in my head, I sat in what felt like a numb coma, trying to remind myself to breathe and calm down. I went from worrying the baby was coming too early to hoping the contractions would dissipate, so I didn't have to make a hospital trip in the middle of our crisis. I prayed, but I doubted it would even be heard.

Thankfully, and miraculously, the baby stayed put, but every time I had a painful contraction, I kept it to myself. Graham didn't need another thing added to the already exhausting pile he was carrying, and I knew it.

That night, the kids slept, but we didn't. We laid in bed wide awake with not a single word to say but millions of thoughts and terrible scenarios on repeat in our minds.

At one point, I had allowed worry to convince me I would probably die from this and so would my unborn baby. It sounds dramatic and impractical now, but at two in the morning, in the middle of our crises, with pregnancy hormones at an all-time high, it was all very real. As I said earlier, I could jump off a cliff without even being near one, and that's exactly what was happening.

The next morning, we sat in a strange motionless shock in our living room. We had no idea what to do, so we just stayed frozen in fear, saying silent prayers for things to work out and in disbelief that they would.

Graham broke the silence and told me again that we would be okay. Again, I didn't believe him. I wanted to, but I really didn't. Instead, I believed my fears, and as I entertained them, I watched Graham jump up and sprint downstairs to our basement washroom to entertain his own fears. He didn't believe his words, either.

What followed was a sound I will never forget. My usually level-headed, calm husband, the one who has helped hold me together so many times, the one who is solid when I can't be, completely crumbled to the bathroom floor and screamed. His frustrated scream then turned into the sound of him throwing up. The pressure had pushed us both to our breaking points.

The days and weeks that followed are a complete blur to me. They are truly some of the worst, most exhausting, and loneliest days I've ever lived. Neither of us were sleeping. I forced myself to eat, knowing my baby needed the food, but I had no appetite. Graham didn't eat at all. We were both more stressed than we'd ever been in our lives, and we had to navigate through the intensity of hurt feelings, anger, confusion, financial turmoil, and my completely broken heart.

Losing a place where we absolutely enjoyed doing what we do, not being able to see all the clients and staff we loved, and not knowing where our next paycheck would come from to feed our family was devastating and terrifying.

Remaining calm to prevent the early delivery of my third son was one of the hardest things I've ever had to do. I couldn't exercise, which had been my healthy outlet for relieving stress. Instead, I spent countless nights in a hot bath to relax and fight through worry.

I wanted to have faith that we would get through this challenge, but I struggled with not being able to see the way. At times, I wondered where God was. I wanted to trust it would all work out, but I battled so much doubt at the same time. Every night, I fought worry. Harder than all of that was getting up the next day exhausted and empty and trying to be happy and healthy for my boys.

The most challenging struggles are often the ones we go through alone, behind closed doors, with no help or support from our loved ones. Graham and I were broken, but to almost everyone else who knew us, we seemed fine. We pretended to be happy for our kids and our loved ones, but under the surface, we were desperate, sad, frustrated, and angry that this had happened to us. We simply had to get up every day and soldier on despite not having any energy to do so.

Have you ever encouraged others while you desperately needed encouragement yourself? Have you ever given to others when it was you that needed to be given to? Have you ever helped others when it was you that needed the help most?

This was what we did. We smiled over it. We gave through it. We got up again and again even though we didn't even believe that we had any shred of energy left in us to do so. We had to. We had no other choice. There were two precious boys relying on us to get up and a third one on the way, so that was the only option we had.

We both prayed for direction and provision, and although at the time we couldn't necessarily see it, in hindsight, God absolutely held us in His hands through this struggle.

Every day, our needs were met, and every day, we had each other to lean on. God kept us sane and healthy and together. The Bible says, "In him all things hold together." (Colossians 1: 17) This was definitely the case for us. We maybe didn't know it yet, but God was with us in this storm.

Sometimes, we feel alone in the struggle, but that doesn't mean that we are. Our feelings are not facts regardless of how loud they can yell. Mine were screaming louder than ever. It felt bleak. I can't even put into words how broken and empty we both were. I can't even describe the feeling of hopelessness that came as we sold off household possessions to get through another month and watched as our life savings shrunk. I can't even explain how much I missed the gym and all the people I loved so much. But I can say that we made it through, and not only that, we came out better because of it.

Our marriage was better, and our gratitude for each other was deeper. We had more compassion for others who face financial challenges and a much greater love for those who supported us in the ways that they could. Above all, our faith grew. We believed more than ever that God is with us and will provide for us no matter how bleak it all looks because, even though we questioned his presence at times, his provision was undeniable. He was with us.

Sometimes, it takes going through a hard time to see why the steps prior to it were taken. It is only now, many years later, that I can look back and see the provision God had already made for us just one year before all of this had happened.

Let me take you back a year and a half before the gym was sold, and you'll see what I mean. I'll rewind for a moment to when we only had one child, and the second boy was on the way but not yet here. Graham and I had decided we wanted to send our first son to a private school that aligned with our Christian values.

We had prayed about where we were meant to move, and though we didn't know where yet, we listed our house for sale, knowing that it was time for us to relocate. One Saturday afternoon, we went for a drive to the city. It was a drive we enjoyed doing together, and it was a drive we had done many times before.

Being so familiar with the route makes it the strangest thing that, on the way home, Graham took a wrong turn, and we ended up on a road that had a Christian school at the end. We both sat at the stop sign wondering what town we were near because we both knew it was where we were meant to move. We also both knew in that moment that this was the school our son was supposed to go to, and God had answered our prayers and led us directly to it. Literally!

Graham never gets lost. Me? All the time. But Graham has an incredible sense of direction, and knowing this made us know with everything in our hearts that it was a God moment we had just experienced.

We turned left and headed into the unknown town, and as we did, I saw a building on the right-hand side that I knew would be a future location of a second fitness centre. I pointed it out to Graham and shared what I was feeling, and his response was quick, "No, let's not get into a second business." But somehow, I knew in my heart we would have one.

We discovered the town we were near was Listowel, and we knew we needed to move to it. This meant moving out of the town we had lived in for many years, and it also meant a forty-minute commute to the gym we loved running. We did it because we felt it was the right direction for us and our family. It was amazing how everything came together for it to be possible.

We found a great home by a park in a wonderful community and enjoyed the forty-minute commute to and from work to run the gym. We also enjoyed the adventure of exploring a new town and meeting new people. Because the private school had a tuition fee, we both knew we would need to make more money to afford it.

Our first step was to go back to school for business so we could learn how to properly run a business. Our next step was to sort out how to make some additional revenue to fund the private school. We prayed, and we trusted God would lead us, and he did.

Graham had the idea to start a bootcamp in the park up the road from our home as a way of meeting people and adding a bit of additional revenue to fund the extra cost of the private school.

It was a side gig at first. In early mornings and a few evenings, Graham would lead fitness classes we called "bootcamp" at the park near our home. During the day, we ran the gym. Life was good. The bootcamp was growing. The gym was growing, and we were balancing both well, along with our growing family.

As the winter approached, we were faced with the challenge of what to do next. We wanted to continue to work with all of our amazing clients who had been coming to the park. We didn't want to leave them hanging, and we depended on the additional revenue, so Graham brought them into our unfinished basement to keep things going.

This worked well through the winter. Then, the next spring, we carried on outside, and as word spread, more clients joined in. As it grew, we began praying about what the next steps were with this side gig because our unfinished basement wasn't an ideal space. It had cement floors, an open ceiling, and insulation hanging out in some places. We were thankful for it, but we knew it wasn't a long-term solution.

One Sunday, we were listening to T. D. Jakes, a preacher we enjoy. He was telling the story about the widow with the oil. She needed to pay her taxes and didn't have enough money to do it. The tax collectors wanted the money, and if not, they wanted to take her sons as slaves. The prophet Elisha came to her and asked her what she had. She told him a few jars and some oil. He told her to borrow jars from the neighbors and start pouring whatever oil she had into the empty jars. Despite not having very much oil, a miracle happened. As she poured, all the jars were filled to overflow. She then sold the oil, paid the tax bill, and saved her sons. God made a way.

While he was preaching about this, he kept saying repeatedly, "The answer is in your house. The answer is in your house." The premise was that we all have something to offer, something that God has provided that we can pour out. After he had repeated it at least five times, it was as if someone had taken mine and Graham's head and banged them together.

We both got the message loud and clear at the same time. Graham and I looked at each other and immediately knew the answer to funding our sons' schooling and keeping the park workouts going was to renovate our basement into a fitness studio and open an after-hours business in our house.

Our oil was our ability to get people excellent fitness results. The jar was our home, and all we needed to do was start pouring. So, we did. We ran the gym during the day and came home to evening classes, clients, and consultations in our very own finished basement fitness studio. I would put the kids to sleep while Graham led sessions and vice versa.

This went well for a while, but as our family grew and our side gig grew, we knew we needed to have our home space back. A local window company had gone out of business and needed a tenant to sublease the space from them in the exact building I had pointed out to Graham.

Despite my being very nervous about the additional cost this would incur for us, Graham had massive faith that if we rented the space, more clients would come to support the vision we had for fitness, and it would thrive. I believed him because I knew God had pointed that building out to me.

It was February when we got the earth-shattering phone call. Our side-gig business wasn't making much money at that point. In fact, it was just paying the rent and barely managing an administrator and one coach we had just hired.

When we got the news, we did not know how this would work for us, but we knew we had to figure it out. We had to lay off our new staff members, which was so difficult to do, and then we put our heads down and went to work. By May, just a few short months later, it was meeting most of our financial needs. It was nothing short of miraculous. God really made a way where there seemed to be no way.

This was an amazing provision, and I couldn't see it clearly until many years later. Obviously, there was hard work involved too, but I know in my heart that we didn't see what was coming, but God did. He prepared our way so we would have something to provide for our young family.

Most of what we worry about never happens. Home foreclosures, car repossessions, not being able to feed our family, and all the things that I wasted sleepless hours stressing about never even happened.

All the stressing Graham and I had done, all our sleepless nights filled with unimaginable worry was just a waste of our time and energy. What we needed to do instead was trust God. Obviously, that's easier said than done, but this is the lesson I carry with me from this storm and the one I pass on to you. Choose to trust God with your storms. Put more faith in him than you do in your worries.

When we can depend on God, our circumstances may not change, but our state of mind absolutely will. This is how there can be peace in the storm. We can rest when we know we can depend on the one who has the power to calm the storm or see us through it. Either way, we can have peace. It's a choice.

Today, we have multiple businesses—online and brick and mortar. Since losing the gym, we've gained two more. Despite Covid shutdowns, they are doing well and continue to provide for our family. We are grateful to all of our dedicated, supportive clients, staff, and loved ones, and we are grateful that God is always there to meet our needs, even if we don't see exactly how he will do it and even when we doubt if he will.

Pressure turns rocks into diamonds. Breaking points can be starting points if we're willing to keep going and trust, even when it's hard. If you asked me in the thick of our crisis if I was thankful for it, the answer would have been a very fast no. But as I look back and see all the shattered pieces neatly sewn together, I can say that I am thankful, and God is good, and not because it all makes sense, but because he held us when it didn't.

This challenge we lived through was a positive turning point in our lives. It taught us that no matter what happens, we can and will get through it, and it showed us that we don't need to rely on anyone. God gives us just what we need when we need it most. He is our provider, and when we lean on Him, He will make a way where there seems to be no way at all.

There's an expression I love that goes like this: "Rock bottom became the solid foundation on which I rebuilt my life." Sometimes, the tower needs to crumble for us to realize the foundation wasn't solid to begin with. I turned to worry more often than I chose faith. Sometimes, it takes rock bottom to realize that.

The ups and downs of life are a form of strength training, or I should say, faith training. Overcoming our past struggles has strengthened our faith for the ones we face now. The ones we face now will help prepare us for the ones we will face in the future. As hard as they are, we need to understand they are also good for us.

The next time we experience something challenging, we have a reference point to reflect on, a foundation to rest upon, and a reminder that we will get through today because of how we got through yesterday. Sometimes, we have to look back and reflect on all the times we made it through to believe we will make it through whatever we are facing now.

I'm not sure where I would be without faith. I certainly can't imagine facing times like these without it. Having it doesn't stop the storm from coming, but it certainly helps us navigate through it.

To me, it's simple. It's believing that rather than having to take control of every situation, try to solve all the problems and sort out all the answers, we can rest knowing something bigger than us is in control and has all the answers and will lead us through the storm in a way that will have us come out better.

Just because we can't see the air, it doesn't mean it isn't there. We may not see God with our eyes. We may not always feel like he is close, but I believe he is our creator and is with us.

Faith wasn't always a part of my life, but the more I live, the more it has grown in me. Some people have a moment where they suddenly believe there is more to life than what they see with their eyes. For me, that moment came in the form of a car crash when I was nineteen.

I was headed in the wrong direction, not literally, but figuratively speaking, and this life changing moment completely re-directed my steps.

Just a few months after I dove my shiny brand-new red neon off the lot, I wrote it off. I was driving tired because I had pulled an all-nighter at my university home studying for a final exam. I was exhausted but went against my parent's advice to stay the night and drove home instead.

All my roommates had left for a school break, and I didn't

want to stay overnight alone, so instead, I drove the three-hour drive home. I was tired but too young and naïve to even consider how that could affect me.

I was two and a half hours into the drive when the accident happened. The driver behind me said he saw my car cross the middle line a few times before it went all the way over the centre line. I have no recollection of any of this.

I was sound asleep when my car swerved left and over the middle line. Ironically, I smashed headfirst into a rest stop sign and knocked it clean out of the ground. Then my car rolled three times before taking a sudden halt in the side of the ditch, just inches away from a very large tree. Witnesses thought for sure I was dead. The car was so crunched up it was almost half the size it used to be.

I slept through the whole thing. I woke up with glass all over me and the feeling of what can only be described as the biggest, warmest hug. It felt as if someone's arms were wrapped so tightly around me I couldn't move. It felt like a good, tight hug. I felt so much love and no fear at all. I felt safe and completely calm. I had a peace I cannot even explain. I knew something was holding me.

The windshield had shattered all over me. Broken glass was everywhere, and my car was completely destroyed. The passenger side had bent in like a tin can. My new car was mangled, but thankfully, I was okay. I was so relieved I hadn't hurt anyone else.

Three men were standing at the edge of the ditch, and I remember looking up at them and hearing them chat back and forth to one another, contemplating if I would even be alive. I waved to get their attention, and they ran down to me. The door was jammed, and I couldn't get out of the car. As I waited for them to help, I dusted chunks of glass off my legs, arms, and chest. I picked glass out of my hair and dusted it off my shoulders. I looked for blood but saw nothing at all. This confused me. I remember wondering how there could be so much sharp glass and no cuts.

I walked away from the accident without a single scratch

or whip lash. I can't fully explain the change inside of me that happened that night, but I can say this moment awakened a belief that there must be a God who held me tightly and chose to keep me alive that night. I know it to this day.

I know it with complete trust and confidence; that's faith. I can't see it. I can't show it to anyone else. I can't even fully explain it, but there is a certainty in me that could never be taken away.

As a child, I never went to church. It wasn't a part of our lives. Religion had let my mom down in a lot of ways, and so instead of church, my mom told me Bible stories and listened to Christian songs as we drove to our cottage. She taught me how to pray and showed me how to have a relationship with God. Sometimes, I would ask questions, but most of the time, I would just listen curiously.

I have a very early memory of being afraid at night and having a hard time falling asleep. My mom came in and said a prayer with me and shared how I could ask God into my heart. She explained I would never be alone if He was there. I was maybe five or six years old.

I said a prayer with her, and on the many nights that followed, I remember saying prayers again, hoping someone heard them but still unsure if this God mom spoke of even existed. However, there was a peaceful presence that I hadn't noticed before, and I knew something felt different.

As I grew, I veered away from any desire to hear Bible stories. When I began dating my husband in high school, he often talked to me about God. He grew up going to church regularly. I wasn't open to hearing him because I believed religion was the source of many problems in the world. I had religion and relationship confused. Now, I know there is a big difference.

I knew of God, but I didn't know God until I experienced him for myself. That car accident changed so much for me. Before it, I was a partying university student with no real direction. I drank too much. I got high too often. I showed up to class hungover or, in one case, still drunk from the night before, and I didn't really think about my future. After the accident, I believed my life had meaning and a purpose, and I wanted to discover what that was.

I started reading the Bible a little. I started praying more often, and I developed a desire to know my Creator and His purpose for my life. I had a newfound faith that He had a plan for me, and I began searching for what that was.

In hindsight, I firmly believe God used that car accident to bring me closer to him. I'm not saying he caused it. I don't believe he causes bad things to happen, but I am saying he uses everything—both good and bad—to bring us closer to him. The Bible says, "All things work together for good to those who love God and are called according to his purpose." (Romans 8:28) I believe this wholeheartedly.

It doesn't say that bad things won't happen, but it promises that even if they do, there will be good that comes from them.

There's a story in the Bible about a wise man and a foolish man. Both the wise man and the foolish man faced hard times. Neither were exempt. The difference was not the size of their house, the strength of their house, or the materials their house was made of.

It didn't matter who had more money or social media followers, or who was better looking. All that mattered was what was underneath the house. The difference was their foundation. One stood solid on the rock, and one wavered on sand.

One sat on something so stable that no matter what happened, the house could not be moved. The other sat on something so unstable, it easily fell.

The parable says that the rain came down, the streams rose, and the winds blew and beat against both of the houses. The one built on sand fell with a great crash. The other remained standing.

Jesus is the rock in this story. Without him, the house will crumble. Without a belief in our Creator, without faith in something bigger than us, we can lose purpose, hope, stability, and even protection.

When life gets shaky, we either shake with it and crumble, or we cannot be shaken at all. We either worry, or we choose to rest. Being solid through the storm is supernatural. The house on the rock stands solid, with a peace that surpasses all understanding. Without faith, it's very difficult to remain standing through all of life's many trials.

Without faith that things will be okay, I would worry instead. Without faith that God has me and my loved ones in his hands, I would worry about them constantly. Without faith that things will work out, I would worry they wouldn't. But because I have faith, I can rest knowing that even if I don't know the way, there is one. Even if things don't go how I'd like them to, they will work out.

Worry stole my ability to live. Faith allows me to live again. Worry says, "What if?" but faith says, "Even if." Even if something bad does happen, even if the circumstances are awful, I won't face them alone, and I will get through it and come out better.

It may not work out perfectly or how I wanted it to, but it will absolutely work out in a way that is good for me. I can rest knowing that. I can choose to trust rather than choose to fear, and that choice allows me to live with peace rather than anxiety.

Don't get me wrong. This choice is not an easy one. Sometimes, the absolute worst things can happen, and rather than choose faith, we are tempted to look at the circumstances and let them overtake us, but making the harder choice will allow for us to rest amidst the hardest of challenges.

All of this is easy to say and so much harder to live out. I am coming through a season of that harder part as I write this. My husband and I recently lost one of our very best friends. In fact, I would call him a brother instead. He was thirty-three years old and left his four incredible young children and their beautiful mom to carry on this life without him in it.

Graham and I were devastated and so were all the wonderful

friends and family who know them. It was tragic. He was playing with his kids in the water at a cottage, and they came to shore, but he didn't. The reasons for such a tragedy aren't clear, but what is clear is that life continues without him here, and that's the hardest part because life without him certainly doesn't feel like life to those he left behind.

When something happens that doesn't make sense and doesn't seem right or fair in our eyes, we can easily begin to question everything we believed, and that's exactly what I did during this tragedy. Others did as well.

Some people who are close to me asked questions like, "How can you still have faith after this?" "If there is a God, why would he let this happen?" and "I just don't think your God is love. How could love take a good man away from his family?" I pondered these questions, and others, as well.

A few months after his death, while I was driving to get some space for myself, I discovered I was angry at God and hadn't even known it. My music shuffled as it sometimes does, and a song came on my playlist that I hadn't chosen. It was a Christian song called "Rescuer" by Rend Collective. I usually love that song, but that day, I wasn't in the right head space to love it.

Every time the singer repeated, "He's our rescuer," I could feel the fury in my soul rise. The anger that had been raging over my sadness began to make its way to the surface.

I quickly pulled over. I ferociously turned off the song, slamming the button as hard as I could, and just as I did, I could see that my hands were shaking. That's the moment I realized I was about to explode. I opened my mouth, and the volcano erupted. "You call yourself a rescuer? You're a fake! A fraud! Where were you, rescuer?"

In mid scream, I was interrupted by my phone ringing. I tried to end the call, but my finger missed the button and accidentally accepted the call. I took a breath, faked a calm voice, and forced out, "Hello."

It was my mom. She skipped the hellos and went right to her reason for calling, "I felt I needed to call you right away. I need to tell you Alison; God mourns this loss with us. He is sad with us. The God you love does not cause bad things like this. He is good, and he is sad right there beside you."

I cried and shared how I had been in the middle of a yelling fit. She said she had suddenly felt she needed to call me and tell me that. I took a breath and told her I would call her right back. I needed a few minutes to process what had just happened.

When I hung up the phone, it was as if all my anger had melted away, and under it was a deep sadness for four special little people and their precious mom.

When she said He mourns with us, I realized I was angry at God for something He hadn't done. Though I still don't understand why God didn't intervene on that day and rescue our friend from drowning, I did know that God is good; God is love, and I needed to choose faith in this very hard time.

When we don't understand something, our brains try hard to fill in the gaps. Thinking God caused this was a false leap. Sometimes, we can let anger take over, and we can jump too far on the other side or throw out all the good stuff along with the bad.

Sometimes, our beliefs can be shaken and that shaking can either get us to choose doubt and fear, or it can allow us to decide even if. Even if we don't know why, we still believe God is good. Even if it didn't go the way we desperately wanted it to go, we still know God loves us. Faith is knowing it will somehow still work out, and it's trusting He sees the bigger picture we don't see yet. It's leaning not on our own understanding, and that is so hard, but that is choosing faith and is so much easier than stressing and worrying.

We live in a world where bad things happen to good people. We live in a world where people make choices and mistakes, and these have consequences. We live in a world that isn't perfect, but it's temporary and one day, we will see perfection when we arrive in Heaven. Until then, we hold on to faith.

Faith says even if it doesn't go as we wanted it to, we can trust that He is God and we are not, and this realization has brought with it an incredible peace. I'm still very sad for my friend and her kids and for their loss. That sadness will probably always be there in some capacity because it's a sad thing that happened.

In the same breath, I am also at peace that I don't see the bigger picture yet, and the God I love does, and He promises us that He works "all things for good." I'm certain we will see good in all of this, and I look forward to that part of this sad story. It doesn't mean we don't have questions or even doubts, but it means we can have faith even with those questions and doubts.

A good friend shared with me you can doubt and have faith at the same time. They can co-exist. Just because you have doubts, it doesn't mean you don't have faith. This perfectly described how I feel. It reminded me of the story of the man who wanted to be healed, and Jesus told him to just believe. The man's response was, "I do believe, Lord, but please help my unbelief." It's okay to have both.

During our grieving, another friend told us that faith is like a muscle; the only way it gets stronger is if it's exercised. The way that happens is by facing the struggle rather than avoiding it and choosing to trust rather than choosing to fear.

Without struggle, we can't strengthen our faith. I know he's right. Though I certainly don't wish for the struggle, in fact, I would much rather avoid it entirely. I also know there is something so powerful about it, and what we gain when we can fully embrace it rather than resist it is incredibly valuable. The shaking has made my faith even stronger.

Though this has challenged my faith, it has strengthened it all the more. I believe there is a heaven, and one day, we will see him again. I believe God has a plan and a purpose and will be with us through the hard parts. Faith is refined and perfected in the fire.

It's the most important pillar in my battle against worry because I can rest knowing that the object of my faith is God, and therefore, I don't have to have all the answers, and even when things don't go my way, He is still with me.

Just a few months after our friend died, my father passed away as well. He was 82 and had been battling ALS for several months. When he got the official diagnosis, I prayed for God to heal him. I desperately wanted him to live. What happened instead was my dad turned his heart toward Jesus.

He began watching preachers on television, reading the Bible and praying, and believing there was more to life than what we see. He didn't want to die, but he absolutely knew where he was going when he closed his eyes on this world. That faith carried me through the sadness of losing him. Knowing this brings me peace and comfort. I can't see heaven with my natural eyes, but I have faith that one day, I will.

I am far from perfect. I'm not always strong. I struggle with my faith, and I don't have it all together. I make mistakes, little ones and big ones, too. I have hard days. I don't have all the answers. I still doubt even though I have faith. In fact, I doubt a lot—more than I wish I did. And some days, I still crumble. But faith allows me to keep getting back up, no matter what.

I get back up because I know God has a purpose for my life. I get back up because there is a reason I am still here. I get back up because three beautiful boys and so many wonderful people love and support me, and I love them back. Together, we encourage one another to keep going. We are called to run the race with perseverance, and that's what I choose to do.

When I shared some of these past struggles with a friend of mine recently, she asked me how I was okay through it all, and more than that, "still help and inspire so many others along the way."

I could have told her so many things; I could have said Graham gets me through, or my kids do, or my loved ones, my career, my athletic goals, or my writing passion.

All would have been valid answers to how I keep getting back up, but none would point in the right direction because God is the reason I can get back up through it all.

Not religion. Not condemnation. Not rules or standards or giant expectations that I could never live up to. Instead, a belief in something bigger than myself and a relationship with the one who created me.

We are not just physical beings. We are spiritual too, and what connects our spirit to our creator's spirit is love. Love binds us like glue because He is love. Having a relationship with the love that created all things is a beautiful gift.

He loves regardless of skin color, gender, sexual orientation, past mistakes, future mistakes, and present ones, too. He doesn't care what you've done. He doesn't care who you know, or how many letters follow your name or don't, how many good things you've done, how many bad things you've done, or how many zeros come after the number in your bank account. He loves you on your very worst day, and that love is an unconditional, no-matter-what kind of love.

If you let him, he will see you through whatever storm you have been in, and every other one to come after that, just like he did and does for me.

I hope you can examine your faith and establish a foundation that is solid, one that will see you through any storm. For me, that is Jesus.

What I have learned is that I need faith every day because when I am weak, He is strong, and I am weak a lot. That's a fact. I'm more thankful than ever to have faith because the storms that shake us to our core will never crumble us when we have the creator as our foundation. Love always protects.

My belief is not condemning; it's not a dictatorship of rules. It's freeing.

Whatever the storm, nothing can ever separate us from His love for us.

I don't know all the details of how He works, but I know that when we give our lives to Him, He will see us through every storm, even the worst ones we cannot imagine finding a way out of.

So, that's where I point, yesterday, today, and tomorrow, to a love that's bigger than the storm ever could be and in the direction that is right for me. The good news is that you can also discover a newfound peace with a faith that, no matter what is shaking around you, cannot be shaken within you.

It doesn't have to be anything fancy, just decide to live in a state of even if rather than what if. Decide to trust God rather than put trust in fear, worry, or doubt. Decide to seek your purpose on this earth because there is a reason you are here, and when you discover it, you'll live life to its absolute fullest, and that's the life you deserve.

Faith is the reason I have peace when I should have fear. It is what has helped me overcome this worry-fest that used to party in my brain, and it is something all of us can discover. A life with faith is a life that doesn't have to know worry because worry says what if, but faith always says even if, and it gives us the strength to get up even if we don't know how.

I think religion complicates what was always meant to be so simple. My children recently showed me this. Andrew loves his little brother Zachary, but as you've been learning, more often than not, he also loves getting under both of his brother's skin.

We were sitting together finishing lunch when Andrew picked up a blue pencil crayon and joked, "Let's write out all the bad things Zach has done."

I asked him, "How would you like it if all of your mistakes were written out for all to see?"

He shrugged as if he wouldn't care and then wrote on the notepad, "Zach is bad."

I immediately gave him the stop-it-now mom glare, and he set the pencil down. Zach quickly picked it up and defended himself by scribbling out what had been written. I knelt down beside him and looked him in the eyes and said,

"That's exactly what Jesus did for us. He scribbled out all of our sins because he loves us."

Then I used the pencil and wrote the truth: "Zach is good, loved, acceptable, perfect, pleasing, and righteous."

He smiled and asked me, "What if I scribble out all the good things about me?"

The words jumped out of my mouth, "You can't. You are His creation, and creation can never undo what the creator has done." At that point, all three of my sons surrounded me with smiles, affirmed by God's love for them.

It's that simple. John 3:16 says, "For God so loved the world that he gave his one and only son, and whoever believes in him shall not perish but shall have everlasting life."

He loved us so much that he made a way for us to be with him forever, and not only that, we can be with him today. Having a relationship means we don't have to wait for heaven to live free. It means that we can have freedom right now.

The relationship we can have with our creator is simply one of love. He loves us so much that he doesn't want us to ever have to worry. He died so we could be free from a life of fear and worry, and all we have to do to have this freedom is believe. It's that simple.

Instead of laying in bed sleepless allowing the worry reel to rob my peace and ruin all the beauty of what is, I can set all the worry aside and choose to enter the peace of knowing that no matter what happens, I will always be okay.

"Do not worry about tomorrow." Mathew 6:34 was a command Jesus gave his disciples, and it used to be one of the biggest challenges for me to follow. *How can I not worry about tomorrow when today is falling apart? When my father is dying, and my friend is mourning, and what we love dearly has been ripped from us? How can I not worry about tomorrow when today looks so bleak?* I can choose not to. It's that simple. Whenever I veer toward worry, or am tempted to consider what if, I allow it to be a reminder that my trust isn't in the right place, and I refocus on putting my trust in God. Choosing faith is so much better than choosing worry.

Even if tomorrow looks bleak, God will never let me go. I can rest knowing that I am loved, safe, and always looked out for, and so can you. That is the promise we can hold on to, and as we feed this fire, worry fizzles away, and everlasting peace consumes its place.

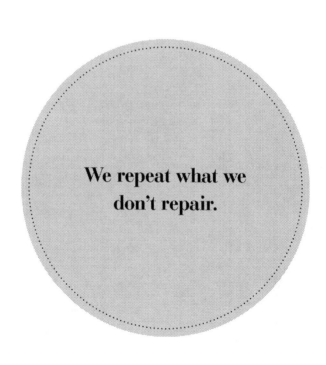

We repeat what we don't repair.

Inner Work

Inner work is something I approach prayerfully. The work is done by God as we lean on him to walk us through healing from all the traumas and trials we have faced. As his word says, "God who began the good work within you will continue His work until it is finally finished on the day when Christ Jesus returns." (Philippians 1:6) We won't be finished until the perfect time, but we can trust that he will complete the work.

In order for healing to begin, we need to be willing to go back to some places that maybe don't feel very good to revisit but need to be faced to fully heal and move forward.

It wasn't until recently that I learned where my worrying habit began. Discovering the root has been monumental in removing worry from my life. Yanking the weed out by its root is the only way to ensure it'll never grow back, so it's important we do the digging necessary to be free. Like many deeply rooted habits, mine began in my childhood.

I used to think healing your inner child was silly, but then I discovered firsthand the impact that childhood trauma can have on our ability to parent. As I dug, I learned it can also affect everything else.

For years, I've hated noise. I never knew why. I never even thought to question why. I simply accepted this as a part of who I am; I'm a person who doesn't like noise. That was my story. And it worked for a little while. That is, until I became mom of three young boys and owner to a tiny and slightly barky, but very cute, Yorkie named Daisy. The noise that would naturally accumulate with a full house created constant tension for me, but I didn't have the awareness of why because I always felt so tense.

That is, until the noise woke me up. My boys were arguing, as they often do. This is the nature of three boys so close in age; they don't always see eye to eye, and being referee is a role I've taken on without even knowing it. It's also one I am working on letting go.

The argument began because of a toy. Someone found a Beyblade under the couch. All three wanted to claim it as theirs. We are still working on sharing and communicating and probably will need to for many years to come. Some days, I genuinely feel as if I'm on repeat and hope eventually my efforts will sink in. Until then, it's all a work in progress and far from perfect.

It happened so fast. My oldest said it was his. The other two were ready to pounce and claim it as theirs, and they did. They jumped into a tug of war for the toy, and I could feel the tension building in my body. It escalated right alongside the noise. The louder they got, the more suffocated I felt.

I hate yelling, and I could feel my entire body tighten as the argument escalated. I cringed and covered my ears, and then, without even thinking before I acted, I intervened by screaming, "Stop fighting! Stop fighting. I hate your yelling!"

It was loud. It was so loud it scared me. It sounded and felt like a roar, and it scared them, too. My youngest was startled from fear and looked up at me with his already big eyes even bigger. His lip quivered as if he was about to cry. No one said a word, and they all stood frozen.

This wasn't the first time my words had come from a place deep within my soul. I completely overreacted again. The violence that came out of my mouth came from a place that was buried deep inside of me, and I was afraid of it because it made me feel out of control.

Thankfully, my husband intervened much more rationally. He rarely raises his voice and almost never matches their energy. Not much gets him rattled. Sometimes, I wish it would, but he's the solid calm our family needs.

In this case, it was good he didn't get rattled. Instead, he put the fire out like a mature adult. He separated the boys and took the Beyblade away, and of course, everyone calmed down.

Everyone except for me. Even afterward, that feeling of not being able to breathe or drop my shoulders down was one I couldn't shake. I knew I needed to take some space for myself to relax. Thankfully, I've gotten much better at being aware of what I need.

I told my husband I wanted to go for a drive, and he understood. What he and I hadn't understood over the previous nine years was why noise made me feel like I was suffocating.

I hadn't connected the dots yet. That is, until I went for that drive.

As I drove down country roads lined with big trees, I watched the sky change pink in preparation for a beautiful sunset, and I prayed. I asked God why I have such a difficult time with noise. Even happy noise sometimes produces a stress response in my body. I'm so aware of the tension I hold when it's noisy.

Within a few seconds of that prayer, it all came rushing back to me. I had a memory from my childhood. I was laying in my bed with my ears covered with my hands. My response to noise is the same today as it was when I was little. Yelling at my boys to stop fighting is exactly what I would yell to my parents when I was a child.

If you had asked me ten years ago if my childhood traumatic, I would have told you absolutely not. I had two parents who loved me. All my tangible needs were met. I had siblings, friends, and more than I could ever ask for. But I didn't see the trauma that was there because I hadn't done the excavating yet.

When we dig, we see what's been underneath the surface all along. And what's under the surface will absolutely affect the quality of life above it, even if we aren't fully aware of how. Even if it's difficult, it's important to do the digging.

My parents did the best they could raising five children, facing a challenging bankruptcy head on, and starting what later, with my brother, became a multimillion-dollar business. On top of all that, my mom carried a career as a registered nurse for over thirty years and then followed her heart on a preventative health frontier, opening the gym I ran. I can imagine life was busy for them and certainly not easy.

My parents' entrepreneurial spirit and heart for helping others inspired my career path as a health and fitness entrepreneur with a deep desire to serve others and improve their quality of life. I love my parents to my core. However, just like me and all parents, they weren't perfect.

Many nights, too many to count, I fought to fall asleep while they fought each other. I don't recall the details of their arguments, but I remember the noise. To an adult, their conflict may not have been so scary, but as a child, I look back and remember it feeling ferocious and terrifying.

Almost every night, I laid my head on my pillow to the sound of screaming and yelling. I would cover my ears with my hands or blanket or my stuffed Mr. Bear, sometimes all three, to drown out the constant back-and-forth arguing. My entire body would tense, and no matter how hot I got under it all, I stayed put, hoping they would stop.

Sometimes, I would bring my head out to yell down to them, "Stop fighting! Stop fighting! I hate your yelling!" I screamed it as loud as I could, but it was never loud enough to be heard.

Many times, their arguments mounted to an emergency exit by one of my parents. I would listen as doors slammed, and then I would watch from my bedroom window as one of them, usually my mom, got in the car and drove away into the darkness. Afterward, I would return to my bed, cry, and worry my mom was gone forever.

I was too young to process all that had unfolded but old enough to worry that my mom may never come back. Watching her leave was the beginning of so much worry for me.

I realized as I drove and reflected after my boys Beyblade debacle that this was where it all began. I would lie awake crying and worrying, some nights frozen with fear at the thought of never seeing her again. Since those scary moments, waves of worry smashed over me almost daily, and it became normal for me to stress about little, and big, things.

Lack of sleep became something that was normal for me as well. From as early as I can remember, maybe age seven until age eleven or twelve, I would sneak into my parents' room in the middle of the night, after the fights were long over, and find a place in between them to sleep.

When I grew too big to fit in the middle, I would lie on the floor beside their bed. Some nights, I would even squeeze under their bed so they couldn't see me. This way, they wouldn't force me back to my bed.

If they caught me, I would tell them I was scared, and I was, but now I know I was also checking to make sure my mom had come back home. I couldn't sleep until I knew they were both there.

Almost to this very day, I have felt the same way when my husband goes away. I've spent years working at being able to fall asleep when he isn't with me. The more I've learned to trust God and let go of fear, the better it has gotten, but it has taken time to work through this.

I know I was too young to understand it all, but I also know I was old enough to let worry become a pattern in my life. The very worry I would struggle years to escape from began in those fragile early years filled with noisy, sleepless nights.

Though many of the nights muffle in my memory, some nights stand out vividly, and as I drove, I allowed myself to face them because inner work is about allowing yourself to go to the hard places you'd rather not revisit, so you can heal from the pain inflicted. Knowing God is with me as I go there gave me the strength to do it.

Years later, when I was in university, my parents went through what I now know to be a healthy separation. At the time, though, it was traumatic for me. We want our parents to be together even if it's unhealthy, and learning they may not always be together was extremely difficult for me.

They took a year and worked through a lot of their challenges. Since their time apart, they get along much better. I'm thankful they worked at things. I'm thankful to have had two parents who loved each other enough to fight harder for their marriage than they did with each other. And, though I am thankful, I regret they didn't work at it all much sooner in their marriage, before they had kids.

If my mom and dad had done the inner work necessary to heal from their childhood traumas, I know they would have parented and behaved much differently. We can't force others to do this work, but we can be the first to break the cycles created by those who haven't.

We owe it to our children and ourselves to excavate, to dig deep down into the foundations of our lives and ensure that all the cracks have been filled, and in some cases re-pour a new foundation if the old one isn't stable.

If we don't do this inner work, we will play out our trauma patterns for the rest of our lives and likely pass on more to our children. Breaking the cycle will set everyone free. The best way to do that is to go back to the painful places in our lives and spend time examining them. Dig into them by questioning what beliefs were formed as a result and then allow God the chance to heal us where we maybe haven't done so yet.

Unfortunately, though, too many adults prefer to blame others for the mess in their lives and hide all their issues rather than face them head on. Some are afraid to let themselves go there. Some are afraid to look at it all because the pain of doing so is much too great. Some have covered it all over for so many years they truly believe they are fine and lack the awareness that the cycles and patterns in their life happen because they have unhealed trauma.

Some even think they've dealt with the mess of their childhood when really, they've just hidden it. The truth is, as I recently realized while cleaning my son Andrew's room, a mess is still a mess in the closet.

Andrew is a messy genius. Let me explain the genius part first; I'm not just saying he's a genius because I'm his biased mom. I genuinely believe this because I've witnessed his mind in action. When he was two and a half, he dismantled the child proof doorknob that even I couldn't figure out, handed it to my husband, and asked to go play outside.

When he was five, he created a fully functional Beyblade and launcher out of Lego blocks and then explained how the gears worked. He's nine as I write this and can create almost anything. His latest invention was a Spiderman web shooter that shoots a magnet attached to a string across the room from a watch. He has etched a spider and spider web designs all over it. It's a scientific work of art that my mind cannot even fathom. Somehow, he made it work.

A recent breakfast conversation started with him telling me, "Mom, I changed my mind about the electromagnetic shield. I want to make a repulser instead." I have no idea what a repulser is, or an electromagnetic shield, for that matter. When I asked him what they are, he replied very matter-of-factly, "It's a small energy cannon that fits in my hand, and when I press the button, it shoots like a laser. It's highly explosive, but don't worry, I would never use it for bad. I would protect myself with it and hit targets." This is an example of a very typical conversation with my son Andrew.

He is always dissecting how things work and contemplating what his next invention will be. He often asks if he can take our computers, cell phones, remotes, and almost anything electronic he can get his hands on apart to see what's inside. His mind fascinates me and simultaneously drives the lover-of-all-things-clean side of me nutty.

I said he is a messy genius, so let's get to the messy part of that equation. His room is a disaster on a good day. It's not the lived-in-look kind of messy. It's the where-is-your-floor kind of messy. Despite not being able to see the floor, he knows exactly where everything is located on it. If I clean it, he loses things. How this makes any rational sense, I do not know, but that's okay. I've learned not to rationalize his genius mind. No one needs to fit into my box; he has his very own.

Because I dislike clutter, but equally respect how his creative mind works, we recently had a conversation about cleanliness to find a healthy middle ground. We came to an agreement that he would do his best to keep the clutter contained to bins in the closet, but when he was in creation mode, he would focus on cleaning up afterward, no matter how messy it got.

This time, he needed help because it was far beyond messy. It was bordering on hazardous. As I looked at the giant heap in the middle of the floor, I felt overwhelmed by it. I wanted to just sweep the entire pile into the closet without first going through it and throwing out the garbage and cardboard pieces he no longer needed. I had the thought that it would be so much easier to just dump it all in the closet and shut the door. But then I had this realization; a mess is still a mess in the closet.

If I just dump it all in, I'd be keeping the mess but simply moving it, and that would defeat the purpose of this attempted clean up. Then I had a bigger realization; so many adults haven't dealt with the mess of their childhood. Instead, they've swept it all into the quiet corners of their memory closet and shut the door in hopes of never seeing it again.

Some even believe they have dealt with the mess, but unless you've gone back, picked through that pile, healed from the hurts, dealt with the traumas, and thrown out all the stuff that no longer serves you, it's all still there, just waiting until someone or something opens the closet door. When that happens, it can come flooding out all at once as an outburst or, in my case, a feeling of panic, suffocation, and a massive yelling explosion.

It can also rear its head in the way we relate to our loved ones, ourselves, food, money, life stress, and so much more. Our cycles, patterns, habits, coping mechanisms, and beliefs are all influenced by the trials and traumas we haven't yet faced head on. All it takes is getting triggered, and unhealed trauma comes boiling up to the surface.

When we can look at the pain, we can heal from it, but so many would rather circle around it to avoid ever having to go back there. They believe this keeps them safe. What they don't know is that despite their best efforts to be okay, to avoid the pain, to cover it over, or sweep it into the closet, it is affecting them physically, emotionally, mentally, and spiritually.

Unhealed trauma bleeds into our lives in some way or another. If we want to be healed, we need to do the clean-up work required to get there, no matter how painful, uncomfortable, or hard it is. I believe God is just waiting for us to ask Him to come in and show us how to clean it all up. He is the Wonderful Counselor we all need.

It's so important to tackle the hard things now. Otherwise, they will affect the future. Worry is a very hard habit to break. It's difficult to go back and search for the root of where it all began, but in order for the plant to thrive, the weeds need to be pulled out around it from under the surface. If you can grab it from the root, you'll forever be free.

That's what happened for me. I discovered the root. The trauma and damage to my sense of security as a child has impacted my sense of security as an adult. How could it not? As a child, I struggled to find peace amidst the noise, and now, as a mom of three, I also struggle.

I was left with sleep issues, noise issues, and a definite post-traumatic stress response to disagreements of any kind. I was also left with the habit of worry.

I remember downplaying my trauma to a friend who had been through what I considered real trauma as a child. I viewed a little screaming and yelling as just that—little. This view kept me from taking the time to zoom in and consider the implications it may have had on me and my life and the way I respond to my children now.

All that changed when I heard Mastin Kip speak about trauma, and I read his book, *Claim Your Power*. It helped me in so many ways. I learned trauma is trauma, no matter how small. It's not the size or severity that matters, but it's how we process it and how it impacts us and then, how we live it out, that really counts.

Everyone has had trauma in some capacity, and if left unhealed, it will absolutely rear its ugly head in some way. Eventually, the mess in the closet leaks out through the cracks. Something comes along and triggers it, and the reaction doesn't fit the circumstance.

As I drove and reflected on how a hidden Beyblade helped me discover something I had been searching many years to find, I realized that even me going for this drive was significant. Escaping the noise is exactly what my mom and dad did regularly.

With no communication, or sorting through the problem, one of them got in their car and drove away instead. They left the argument without resolution. I was simply modeling what I had witnessed for years. Escaping was their coping mechanism, and at that moment, it was also mine.

So many habits and patterns in my life have been trauma responses to the noise I so badly wanted to escape growing up. I avoided crowds. I hated loud music. I had convinced myself I'm a quiet person and even called myself an introvert; I'm so not an introvert.

I realized that, in doing all the above, I was refusing to let my children work through their disagreements because I couldn't stand hearing the conflict. The irony is amazing. My trauma response to my parent's lack of communication and constant noise was holding my children back from learning how to communicate and work through their disagreements. The bottom line is simple; we live out what we don't face.

I've overreacted to my boys' innocent squabbles so many times. I've coped by escaping, and I've avoided certain people and situations to protect myself. I developed a worrying habit that often caused me more stress but felt familiar and became a default setting for me.

When something tough happened, instead of perseverance and positive thinking, I jumped to *what if* right away, and I lost thousands of hours of sleep, letting my mind race down far-fetched rabbit holes that never end and never ended up happening.

That feeling of suffocation is real and makes so much sense because it was exactly how I responded to the noise as a child. For years, my body has done a full re-enactment of the seven-year-old me, suffocating under pillows, blankets, and Mr. Bear, trying to drown out the noise.

All of these realizations were beautiful and healing, and I let them flow along with the healing tears. I was so grateful to have yet another prayer answered. Discovering the root of my habit is the first step to understanding so much. I knew this would be the awareness I needed to move forward worry free.

As I continued to drive, I watched the clouds move over the sunset I had been expecting, and it slowly began to rain. My tears flowed as the sky unloaded hers. Even nature needs to let it out. God's perfect design was never for us to hold everything in or hold it all on our shoulders. He waits for us to come to him and lay it all down. The Bible says to "cast all your care upon Him." (1 Peter

5:7) When we do this, we relinquish the burden and heaviness, and the lightening of this load frees us from it.

Watching the rain pour down my van window, I realized something amazing; all that we are meant to be, all the beauty we have to share with our loved ones, it can easily be covered by clouds if we don't heal from the weight of our childhood traumas. We need to heal so we can shine, and when we shine, we provide a light for others to heal, too.

Awareness is a powerful weapon. God's word always says it best, "And you shall know the truth, and the truth shall make you free." John 8:32

Knowing exactly where our trauma patterns and reactions began, and what they are, allows us to begin the walk to freedom.

For some, this is a long walk, for others a short one. Either way, one step in front of the other allows us to move forward toward the discovery of who we were always meant to be—before the trauma. Dr Gabor Mate specializes in helping people with trauma, and I love how he puts it: "Every human has a true authentic self. Trauma is the disconnection from it, and healing is the reconnection to it."

When we're willing to do this walk, so much can change for the better. We can be free to be who we were always meant to be, and this can allow the same freedom for our children. Now that I know where worry began for me, I can help prevent the same patterns from starting for my children. I owe it to them to continue this walk.

As I returned home from my revelatory drive, the sun pushed its way back through the clouds to complete its exit, and a beautiful rainbow appeared in the sky. The moment could not have been any more perfect.

As I took in all the surrounding beauty, I knew it was God's assurance that he was the blanket keeping that little girl I used to be safe. He was there even though I couldn't see him, and He always will be.

He is the answer to all the problems we face, and no matter

what, He will always see us through the hard times and over to the other side, where we can reach our hand back and help others through their struggles.

Doing the inner work isn't an easy process. Often when I've felt like I'm healed of worry and traumas, something happens, like the argument my boys had and I discover a new layer to the onion of healing.

Getting to the core takes work, and that work starts with being willing to look at all the challenges we have faced and examine how they have shaped us into who we are and what we do or don't do.

Inner work looks different for everyone, and there is no right or wrong way to do it. It's also not a sprint. It's a marathon with many detours, and it requires patience with yourself.

Do not be hard on yourself. Instead, have grace for all that you are, flaws included. That's the God kind of grace. He loves you, imperfections and all. There will be setbacks, but they can be set ups for future success if you take the time, as I did on my drive, to learn from them.

For me, it's been a difficult and worthwhile journey over the last ten years, and I know I'm still a work in progress and will be until my very last day.

I'm never going to be a perfect mom. I will make mistakes, and so will you. But we can be better moms every day. Progress is what this is all about.

It makes sense to me that to move forward, we need to look back and work through any limiting beliefs and false stories our minds have created.

I believe there are millions of methods of healing, but only one healer. My father used to say, "Jesus healed so many different ways." I think that is still true today. Some people choose counseling, others discover meditation and prayer, others delve into self-help books or discover a passion like running or hiking or mountain biking. There isn't a one size fits all approach; there are many approaches for all different sizes.

For me, it has meant reading, taking trauma courses, getting counseling, praying, discovering the promises given to us in the word of God, journaling, taking space when I need to take it, and going back and listing every traumatic memory, big or small, so I can face it head on rather than living my life avoiding the pain it caused.

How can we move forward if we haven't yet looked at and healed from the past? This takes time, but it's amazing how when you focus on something, your mind will show you what you need to find.

Our brain is a fascinating creation. It has memories we aren't even aware of, but when we ask God to reveal them, the memories will flow. A close friend of mine had no memory of being badly bullied as a child until he wrote things out. Then he recalled a time when a group of young boys, who he thought were his friends, beat him up with sticks. He was bruised and cut and could barely walk home to get help.

Once he could recollect this trauma, he could then work through it in a new way from a safe and healthy perspective. He learned so much. He discovered how it had impacted his ability to trust the friends and co-workers he has now. He realized he wasn't allowing people into his life to the level he could had he trusted them more. He often avoided crowds and didn't trust groups of people. He also always feared that people would turn on him. He learned so much from the discovery of that one memory, and the discovery gave him a new sense of freedom in so many of his relationships. First, he needed to make this discovery. That's where healing begins.

We don't know all the things locked up in that incredible closet we call our brains, but just like memories came to him that he didn't even know he had, the same will happen for you if you ask God to reveal what you need healing from. Sometimes, we don't remember all the details or exactly what happened, but we can still go back and work through feelings we have and beliefs we've formed based on them.

I recently had a similar experience with locked up memories. I was doing a Wim Hof breath meditation and noticed tension and pain in my mid-back. As I tried to concentrate on the tension I was feeling and breathe through it to release it, I felt so strongly that I was just a child when this tension began.

I couldn't shake the thought that I had fallen on my back as a child, and I knew it was traumatic. I tried to remember, but I couldn't recall anything like this having happened. I prayed, and I felt God directing me to call my mom and ask her if she remembers me falling hard on my back. She immediately remembered.

I was seven years old. My dad had just purchased me the most beautiful bike. It was pink and white with streamers on either side of the handle bars and pink spoke reflectors, the ones that made a musical clanking noise whenever the tires moved. It was a little girl's dream.

My mom knew at the time that two friends who lived across the road from me were jealous of my new bike. She saw their reaction when I excitedly showed it to them. The sister was eight and her brother was six. They both immediately made fun of it because it had training wheels on it. They called me a baby and walked away laughing.

My dad wanted me to ride the bike with the extra wheels on until he felt as if I was fully ready for them to be off. I was mortified because I knew I could bike without them and because I cared what my friends thought, so I begged him to take the training wheels off.

He was worried I would fall. I insisted I would not ride my new bike unless he took the training wheels off. He reluctantly removed them, and off I flew, fully able to ride the bike without them.

Everything went well for the first few rides. Then, the two

people who I thought were my friends came running from behind me and ripped me off the back of my new bike. My mom witnessed the entire thing from the living room window of our home and came running out to make sure I was okay. My so-called friends ran away as fast as they could. She could hear them laughing as I laid there on my back, shocked, and barely knowing what had just happened.

From that moment, as strange as it may sound, my body held the trauma. So many trauma specialists believe, "The issue is in the tissue." More research is coming out that this is, in fact, true. That disease, tension, and other ailments in our bodies are often presented because of unhealed childhood trauma.

MRIs of people's brains who have endured traumatic events resembled that of stroke patients. Lesions were discovered in certain areas of the actual brain tissue caused by the trauma itself. Trauma has a physical manifestation in our bodies, and if we do not heal, we will have to deal with the consequences somewhere in our futures.

As my mom shared the story, I remembered the bike and what it looked like, I also remembered begging my dad to take the training wheels off and believing that I could ride without them, but I still don't remember the neighbors doing that to me. Maybe I blocked it out, or maybe I was simply too young to remember all the details.

Sometimes, our brains hold memories from us to protect ourselves, and we only remember them if we are willing to do some serious digging and are open and ready to face whatever we find.

After my mom shared this memory, I returned to the breathing meditation, and I forgave the two kids I thought were my friends. Forgiveness is so important. It frees everyone and helps begin the healing process. It's not always easy to do, but it's always freeing to do it. It frees the other person, and it also frees us.

After I let them go, I breathed through the tension and pain in my back, and it completely disappeared within minutes. It was like nothing I have ever experienced before. I firmly believe that God led me through a physical healing process that day.

Healing doesn't have to be mechanical or methodical. In fact, I think in most cases, healing is an art, and it's simply a matter of being open to trying many approaches and avenues and praying about what is best for you. God knows us better than we could ever know ourselves, and his desire is for us to have healing.

Regardless of the method, trauma certainly needs to be healed from. If ignored, or left forgotten, it will affect every area of our lives, and this includes our physical body. It's so important to heal from it by doing the inner work. This allows for not only better physical health but also better mental and emotional health.

When trauma happens, we often form beliefs because of it. These beliefs become cemented into our psyche and become a part of who we think we are. As I did some digging surrounding my parents fighting and the noise that came with it, I discovered that a belief I had formed when I was a child was that money causes fighting.

As I got older, I tried to avoid discussing money but never knew why until I did this inner work. In my mind, I was avoiding an argument. I thought that discussing money caused disagreements. The younger me decided this; therefore, the older me was protecting herself based on what was decided.

I chose to believe a lot of lies about myself, others, and life because of my worry. I always expected the worst-case scenario and believed wholeheartedly it would happen. I didn't trust people easily, if at all. I had sleep issues and could never fully relax, and I had a physical stress response to noise and disagreements of any kind.

The impact we can have on our children if we don't deal with our issues is big. It's so important to excavate and heal all the areas left untouched, or they will seep out of the closet and into our lives.

You do not have to live a life of worry. We deserve the peace that comes with discovering where it began and then letting it go. It is absolutely possible to have it. Sometimes, it simply takes stopping long enough to examine where things came from, why they are here, and if you even need them at all.

Inner work for me has been a process of being open minded, learning new approaches, and realizing that it's necessary to open the closet and face all the things we would rather sweep into the corners and ignore. It's an inside job, and it's an important one.

I am always discovering something to work on, and so long as we continue to try, we will heal and grow and become healthier versions of ourselves. We're never finished until the day our creator calls us home, but we can rest knowing that we will become all that we were meant to become as we put our trust in the healing hands of God.

What I've learned is that the most challenging things to face are usually the most worthwhile. Growth is on the other side of discomfort. In the words of David Richo, "Our wounds are often the openings into the best and most beautiful part of us."

We'll miss out on some incredible opportunities if we avoid that mess in the closet entirely, so open it wide, be brave, and know that your healing isn't just for you. It brings peace to everyone who needs and loves you, and it comes from your heavenly Father who created you perfect and in his image.

The longer the shelf life,
the shorter your own.

CHAPTER 5

Real Food

By the age of fourteen, I was overweight, asthmatic, self-conscious, and chronically sick with bronchitis, strep throat, and mono. I had allergies, fatigue, and low iron. I hated my body, and I felt awful all the time.

How does someone like this break a Guinness World Record for most chest-to-ground burpees in one hour at age thirty-eight and then set a 12-hour record for the most burpees done by a female team? Allow me to share my journey with you and detail how I went from overweight and always sick to discovering my inner athlete and living a healthier lifestyle.

When I was fourteen, I had no idea that how I felt and looked was directly related to the food I ate. My mom hadn't made that connection either, but she was close to discovering it. She was overweight and overwhelmed and started seeking ways to regain her health.

She had me when she was in her forties, and afterward, found it much harder to get her body back in shape post-baby than it was with the other four kids she had in her thirties. The baby weight accumulated and then the stress of life accumulated on top of that. Couple this with unhealthy food habits and a very sedentary lifestyle and it isn't surprising we weren't the picture of perfect health.

I remember her taking me to an herbal weight-loss clinic. We wanted our weight loss to be like magic. After the initial appointment, we were both disappointed. I was too young for the pills, and my mom's blood pressure was too high for the pills. We wished it could be as easy as taking a pill, but it never is.

Sometimes, it takes a scare or even a crisis to help us realize just how valuable our health is and to teach us that our food really contributes to how we look and feel. This happened to my mom, and because of it, she turned our world upside down for the better.

Discovering a lump on her breast gave her a scare, but it was just the wake up that was needed. It created a healthy momentum for our entire family, and it started her on a path to more education beyond her career as a registered nurse. It also pushed her past wanting a magic pill to create a healthier lifestyle. She was determined to lower her blood pressure and get rid of the lump, naturally.

She took nutrition courses, read hundreds of books, got certified in iridology, and sought chiropractors, naturopaths, and Chinese medicine practitioners. She found vitamin companies, natural skin care products, healthier deodorant, and environmentally friendly cleaning products.

Some of her colleagues called these methods strange and even quackery, but she didn't care; she was a woman on a mission to improve her health. She was willing to do whatever it took to discover it, even if it seemed strange to those around her.

She went against the grain, which in her day meant she brought home vitamins, started juicing, and learned about cleansing the body. She made our meals with more veggies and began integrating healthier foods into our diet like rice and broccoli and onions. She stopped drinking as much alcohol; she stopped eating as much takeout and sugar, and then, as if that wasn't a big enough change, she did something even bigger.

She quit her nursing career of thirty years and opened a preventative health business that encompassed massage, reflexology, and several other alternative health modalities. She was brave.

Out of her tiny store-front named Health Options, she began selling vitamins and educating people on preventative health. I distinctly remember a stranger coming into the store when I was helping her get things set up and telling her she was selling "snake oil." He pointed to the shelf filled with vitamins, omegas, minerals, and natural body creams. She kindly asked him to leave, and he did.

It seems so silly today, writing that someone thought her vitamins were snake oil, but back then, she was doing something so different that not everyone believed it was good.

I've learned that when you're ahead of your time or blazing a trail, some people don't understand where you're coming from. Rather than try to understand, they decide instead that you must be wrong or weird or uneducated when, really, you're just further up the trail with a different vantage point. Therefore, it's so important to keep an open mind and not get cemented into your ways.

My mom tried to bring everyone with her on this get-healthy journey but not everyone wanted to come. Some people thought she was having a midlife crisis, some people thought she was involved in a scam, and some didn't have any desire to get healthier at all.

But some people saw it for what it was and appreciated what she was trying to do. They saw her heart and knew she was trying to help people live healthier lives and prevent disease as best they could. They, too, wanted to be healthier and so they were the people that came with her.

She had been in the medical system for a long time and genuinely loved being a nurse, but she wanted to help people avoid having to end up there. She would always say, "You don't want to end up in the medical system because, when you're there, it's because you are sick. Work at getting and staying healthy instead."

The slogan for her newfound business and passion was, "Take charge of your health," and this was what she taught people to do. Many came to see her and regained their health. Many saw tremendous improvement with diseases they were dealing with. All felt the love she had for each person who came through her doors.

A year after she had made this big change, she took her tiny storefront business one step further and moved it into a space where she integrated a fully equipped fitness facility. She expanded the name to Health Options Fitness and Wellness Centre, and I started working at the front desk of the gym when I was fifteen.

My entire family got better because of it. We all saw health improvements. We all lost weight. We all learned more about our bodies and our health. My asthma went away within a year of these healthy changes. Twenty pounds of excess fat came off my body within a year and a half. Antibiotics were no longer something I was regularly taking. I looked and felt much better. Honestly, I got my life back.

My mom's lump went away naturally, and she gained control of her weight gain. She is almost 80 as I write this and still gets on her indoor cycle bike and treadmill regularly. Until recently, so did my dad. She still takes her vitamins daily. She still eats her veggies. She still seeks preventative medicine and alternative modalities wherever she can. She still tells others about the importance of caring for their bodies. She has her share of health challenges, but I firmly believe that had she not taken the path she did way back then, she wouldn't be here today.

My dad and all four of my siblings live active healthy lifestyles, and so do I. We traded fried chicken, pizza, and prepackaged noodles and powdered cheese for kale smoothies and buddha bowls. We traded sedentary lifestyles for active ones. We traded poor health for great health—all thanks to a mom on a mission.

So, why am I telling you this? For a few reasons, three to be specific. First, your past doesn't have to be your future. You get to decide how you want to feel tomorrow. You can choose to have a healthy future by making wise choices today. The power to live better is completely up to you. God gave us a body, and just as he desires us to be good stewards of all he has given us, I believe he desires us to care for the one body he gave us.

Making these choices isn't easy. The easy choice is always the drive-thru. The easy choice is always the pre-packaged, microwavable, fibreless, five-seconds-and-ready option. The easy choice is the one that's loaded with sugar and saturated fats and makes our tastebuds dance and then crave more. But what we don't always see is that the easy choice at the moment is the hard choice in the long run.

If we choose hard now, we will have it much easier later. Hard is having the kale salad when everyone else is having the chips and dip. Hard is having to dice up the veggies and spread them over the healthier dough to make the pizza ourselves or asking for more veggies and less cheese on the one we order from the store. Hard is saying no to the junk food and deciding you want to feel better tomorrow instead of feeling good for a few minutes right now. Hard is sacrificing now so you can live better later.

Jim Rohn said, "Suffer the pain of discipline now or suffer the pain of regret." I can't write it any better than that. It sums up the food debacle we all face every single day. You can choose to clean up your eating habits and feel better now and tomorrow, or you can choose not to.

If not, then when it all catches up to you, and it will, you may regret that you didn't make the choice you could have, the choice you know is the best one for you. It's maybe not the most delicious one right now, but it's the one with the greatest reward later.

I think that's why it's so hard. We don't see the good consequences of choosing the healthy stuff right away. It takes time and consistency, and even then, we don't always see the benefit. We want the instant gratification of a pill and the melt in our mouth deliciousness of chocolate cake rather than the hard, muscle-burning, sweaty effort of exercise and the crunch of a healthy kale salad. Food choices will pay off one day in the future but require effort and discipline today. The work is worth it, but we don't see it paying off right away, and that's the hard part.

My mom did a very hard thing, and years later, my life is easier because she did that. Years later, my health is better because she did that. Years later, my children's health is better because she did that. Your choice as a mom has the potential for a massive reach, and when you choose hard today, tomorrow will be easier for yourself and everyone you love. Knowing that has to be enough of a driving force to make the right choice. If it's not, then be prepared for a potential wake up call much like the one my mom faced. I certainly don't wish that on anyone, but it is absolutely a natural consequence of choosing to live unhealthy.

Second, I'm telling you this because I want you as a mom to know something amazing; you have the power to change your children's lives forever. Never underestimate what a mom on a mission can do. My mom is the reason my passion for moms is so loud. Moms can move mountains. They can change futures. They can redirect paths. By simply changing their lives, moms can impact all the lives around them, and that's exactly what my mom did.

Before she made these changes, I was on a very unhealthy path. Fitness and nutritious food were not even thoughts in my mind. I knew nothing about them. I know wholeheartedly that because of her choices, I am who I am today; I'm healthier inside and out, and I get to help others live healthier.

The trickle-down effect from my mom's healthy choices had an impact so profound she wouldn't even be able to count the number of lives she had positively influenced directly, and then indirectly through me and everyone around me. Thousands of people have become healthier because of one simple choice made by a mom—to learn how to get healthy and to be brave enough to share her findings with others.

My third and most important point is what you eat matters. It really matters. If you want to change how you feel and look, then just like my mom did and just like I did, you'll need to change what you put into your mouth every single day.

You've heard the expression you are what you eat. It's the truth. If you eat nutrient-dense foods, you'll feel good. If you eat healthy, you'll think clearer. If you eat well, you'll live a better life. Every single thing you consume works to form a brand new you every seven years. If you choose wisely today, that new you will be a healthier version tomorrow. If you don't, then it will not.

Food is the foundation for energy in your body. If you're feeding your body poor quality foods, then you're asking it to do all of its daily tasks with inadequate tools. This translates to your body not being able to do its absolute best because the materials you're giving it aren't good ones.

Imagine not having a hammer to put nails into boards, but having a broken piece of wood instead. You could likely still accomplish the task, but it would be a much more exhaustive process, and it would be difficult to trust the job was done right because it wasn't.

I'm speculating here, but I bet you would never load your child up with as much candy as possible and then ask him or her to go to sleep for the night or to fight off a bad infection. Instead, you would give your child the very best food, so his or her body can do the things it needs to do. The same is equally important for yourself.

You are worth the effort. Your body is worth being cared for in this way. You are an amazing creation deserving of love, and in this case, love in the form of healthy, nutrient dense food.

Now, before I get too far ahead here, I need you to know that it wasn't a magical process for me where my mom came in, threw out the pizza, loaded our plates with veggies, and boom, I never struggled with choosing healthy food again and became the athlete I am today because of it. In fact, quite the opposite. It was hard.

Fifteen years of unhealthy eating patterns are a lot of years. I had some very unhealthy food habits. As with my worry habit, habits are extremely hard to break, and these are no exception.

Before it got easier, it got hard. I went through a process where I really struggled with wanting to be healthy and feel good but also wanting all the pizza, chocolate almonds, and the salt and vinegar chips.

I could go small stretches where I would eat well, but then I would always revert to my younger self and overindulge in all the unhealthy stuff. Then I would try again, start fresh on Monday, refocus, and get back on track.

Sound familiar? Maybe you can relate to the on-again-off-again struggle. It felt like years of this cycle of trying to eat healthy but fighting my tastebuds and my already-cemented-in default setting of just wanting to eat all the pizza and not do the workouts.

When I finished university, I took more nutrition courses. I had already taken fitness and health promotion and the personal trainer's course, but I wanted to learn more. At least that's what I told myself; that was partly true. I wanted to learn more about food, but I also wanted to figure out how to break the cycle I kept finding myself stuck in.

As I learned more, I ventured into the world of fitness competitions and dieting down for photo shoots and stage events. It was essentially the other end of the spectrum. Sure, I lost weight, my muscles were very defined, and I looked like the picture of health, but on the inside, I still struggled with having a healthy relationship with food.

The world of fitness competing was good and not so good for me. It was good because it taught me self-discipline and how to control my food cravings. I became mentally stronger than ever before and learned so much about calculating macronutrients, calories, pairing certain foods together, and timing foods right, all to get the best physical results. I learned how food is tied directly to how our body looks, and at the time, looking good mattered the most to me.

The connection I lacked was how food makes us feel and perform. We need healthy fuel to feel our best and do our best, and though looking good is a nice bonus, it can't be the primary focus to sustain a healthy lifestyle.

The challenge was that I had lived from age nine to fifteen feeling self-conscious and being overweight, and finally, I could enjoy being thin and toned. I was so happy to feel good in a bikini for the first time.

What I didn't learn over the course of those four years was how important feeling good is. I didn't feel good. I looked good, but on the inside, I was tired, hungry, and living on a very strict and rigid eating regime that wasn't sustainable for long-term health. As unbalanced as I was before this, I was still unbalanced, just in the other direction.

Leaving this world behind was one of the best decisions I've ever made. It allowed me to move toward performance-based goals rather than aesthetic ones. Ashley Turner puts it this way: "Once we celebrate what our body does rather than obsessing about how it looks, we appreciate our body as an instrument rather than an ornament."

This is exactly what I did. I ventured into running and training for marathons, half marathons and duathalons. I also got more serious about weightlifting.

I took performance nutrition courses and learned how to fuel my body so it could complete physical tasks like biking fifty kilometres or running ten miles. Then, I got into Crossfit competitions and lifting a barbell and doing pullups and handstands and learned to fuel my body to be strong rather than deprive it to be thin.

Feeling good is directly linked to fueling good, and over the years, with more courses and more experience, I finally found a healthy balance with food—one where I could have the chocolate almonds and salt and vinegar chips and still be healthy and feel good.

I didn't overconsume them anymore or get stuck in a cycle of on again, off again. Having a few snacks no longer caused me to fall off the rails entirely because I wasn't on a particular diet, and so I wasn't falling off of one. I was simply eating healthy and exercising regularly so I could perform well and be healthy.

This shift in my personal food relationship helped me help my fitness and nutrition clients so much better. Over time, it also helped me become the athlete I am today.

I run, bike, lift heavy weights, and do a bit of everything. I focus on how I feel and perform rather than how much I weigh. I keep track of the weight on my bar, not the scale, and I work at having a healthy relationship with food.

I focus on fueling well so I can perform well and feeling good rather than trying to be skinny or fit into a certain size or look good in a bikini. I don't even care what I look like in a bikini. I care most about the fun I have in it, and I have zero concern for what I look like while I'm having it.

I'm so grateful I've been able to come to a place of more balance so I can model that to my children and share that with my clients. It's liberating.

My boys need to see a mom who isn't insecure about her body. They need to see a mom who takes care of her health. They need to see a mom who loves herself regardless of what the number on the scale says.

Though I've learned a ton and can absolutely work with a larger variety of clientele because of the nutrition information I've gained over the years, I've learned probably the most valuable nutrition information possible. It's simple; eat real food.

We overcomplicate nutrition with calories and macros and cycling and fad diets and the latest research, but if you really want to feel good, and look good too, the best advice that I could give is to eat real food. I would follow that up with eat when you're hungry and stop when you're full.

When I say eat real food, what I mean is that if it has a large list of ingredients that you don't know how to pronounce, chances are good that it isn't the best for your body. The body was designed to take food in its natural state, break it down, and use all the valuable nutrients provided as the raw materials for building blocks of healthy cells, a strong immune system, and a well-functioning ecosystem.

An apple is real food. Broccoli is real food. Chicken, fish, eggs, and rice are all real foods. Real food is food without a bunch of stuff thrown into it to make it taste better, last longer on the shelf, or look different from how it should look.

The more real food you consume, the better you will feel because your body can use real food; it recognizes it. In fact, your body needs real food to function optimally. So does your mind.

Depression, anxiety, stress, and worry can all be heightened when foods loaded with preservatives and chemicals are consumed. Nutrient-dense, real food helps keep everything healthy.

Web MD says: "If you eat lots of processed meat, fried food, refined cereals, candy, pastries, and high-fat, high-sugar dairy products, you're more likely to be anxious and depressed. A diet full of whole fibre rich grains, fruits, vegetables, grass-fed meats and fish can help keep you on a more even keel."

Consuming real food matters. It's more important than we even realize. I'm not saying you have to be perfect. I'm not saying you can't have certain food products or candy you love. I'm not saying you need to nix entire food groups either. What I'm saying is that if you can focus on consuming foods close to their natural state, you will be healthier mentally and physically for it.

We overcomplicate nutrition a lot. We get detail oriented and want to know exactly how much, how often, and precisely what to consume. We also tend to over emotionalize food. We use it for so many other things than simply satiating hunger. We feed loneliness, boredom, sadness, pain, excitement, overwhelm, and stress.

Eating better is as simple as eating real food as often as possible. It's as simple as eating when we are hungry, stopping when we are full, and eating to fuel not to medicate or alleviate emotions. It is striving to do our best without beating ourselves up about making choices we wish we wouldn't have made. It's okay to have a snack here and there, but it's not okay to beat yourself up for it.

It's simple. We know it's simply said and harder executed. The payoff is worth the work it takes to overcome food struggles because the payoff is feeling good and living a healthier, energized lifestyle in a body we can depend on. The payoff is also showing our children what healthy food is and how to relate to it positively.

Without adding more to your already full pile, I have to be straight with you and tell you that your food relationship, patterns, and habits will lay the foundation for your children's relationship with food. That's a big responsibility.

No matter how old your children are, I can tell you with absolute certainty that it's not too late to start making better choices. No matter how late in the parenting game you are, your kids are still watching and can be influenced positively by your desire to be healthier and fuel well.

If my mom can completely redirect the course of my life for the better at age fifteen by her choice to live healthier, so can you. And the time to start is now. Not tomorrow, not on Monday, today.

If you would have told the overweight, unhealthy, extremely self conscious, sedentary fourteen-year-old me, who just wanted to take a magic pill to get skinny, that I would break a Guinness World Record for most chest-to-ground burpees in one hour and most burpees in twelve hours with a team, and not even care about skinny, I wouldn't have believed you.

That's because I am not who I used to be. One reason for that is because I became what I saw modeled. I tell my mom tribe that children will be what they see, not what we tell them.

My mom modeled an unhealthy lifestyle when I was younger, so I was on the path to living in an unhealthy body as a result. But all that changed when she changed, and because she did, I did too. At age thirty-eight, I had the opportunity to practice what I preach. Andrew brought home the Guinness Book of World Records from school on library day, and as we sat down and explored the pages in amazement at all the incredible things and people in our world, he asked me, "Mom, can I be in this book too?" I told him, "You can do anything you work for." And then we carried on our exploration.

The next day, I was on my lunch break when my words came back to me. "Children will be what they see, not what we tell them." I felt so strongly that I needed to show my boys that they can do anything they work for rather than simply tell them that.

I like burpees. It's weird; I know. The exercise most people despise is the one that I enjoy. I can't explain it, but there is something I love about the symbolism of laying flat on your stomach and having to use all your strength to get back to your feet as fast as possible. Likely, the metaphor of getting back up every time you get knocked down is one that I've lived through so many times that I've strangely grown accustomed to enjoying it.

Because I love them, I Googled how many burpees had been accomplished in one hour. When I discovered the number was 709, I knew with everything in me that I could do more. Without allowing myself the time to second guess it, I submitted the application to attempt to break the record and went to work.

I was ready because of all the steps I had taken previously to this one. I knew how to fuel for the event, and I knew how to train for it. It wasn't easy, but it was so awesome to show my children what it looks like to set a goal and then work toward achieving it.

With my family and loved ones around me, I broke the record, completing 730 burpees in an hour. When my son Andrew hugged me proudly, he whispered in my ear, "I knew you could do it, Mom." And of course, I melted. He believed in me because I first believed in myself, and I know with everything in me that he will believe in himself because he saw it modeled.

I'm so grateful I got to show my boys rather than tell them. I'm incredibly thankful my body was able and ready to do it and that my boys get to see what caring for our bodies looks like.

You don't have to do an insane number of burpees to live healthier; that's not what I'm saying at all. What I am saying is that we need to model healthy habits if we also want our children to have them because they will become what they see.

Your future self is depending on you. Your children are depending on you, and so are theirs. You can look and feel your best tomorrow by making the hard, good choices today.

Don't make excuses. Don't let your default setting let you dictate your direction. Rise to meet your future self head on and be able to say to her that you did the hard thing so she could live a healthier life today.

Real food is a tool in my toolbox to help me overcome worry, stress, and anxiety, and it can also be a tool for you. It's not always the easy choice, but it truly is worth it. Feeling good feels so much better than feeling unwell all the time.

Sometimes, healthy eating can be expensive and not everyone can afford that. The good news is that there are so many ways around the expense. Frozen veggies are cheaper and are still veggies. Canned fruit is less expensive and still fruit. Starting a garden is an excellent way to save money and build a new appreciation for the growing process. Every small choice adds up. It doesn't have to be big or perfect to be good.

You can have more energy, feel good in your skin, and have a strong body and immune system, and all you have to do is start. Try to make healthier choices by choosing to fuel your body with real food, and one day, you may look back in amazement at the impact your one choice has made on all those around you. You'll never know if you never try.

"Train as if your life
depends on it because
one day it could."

CHAPTER 6

Exercise

Just a few years into our marriage, Graham almost died. The doctor told him that had his heart and lungs not been in the condition they were in, he likely would have.

We were in the thick of our fitness careers, so he was lifting weights, running, playing soccer, and leading indoor cycle classes a few times a week. He was eating healthy and exercising regularly, so he was prepared for a fight he didn't even know was coming. Had he not been ready, his outcome could easily have been much different.

Before this life-changing event, I used to think the quote, "Train as if your life depends on it because one day it might," was cute. I would relay it to my clients to give them some extra motivation during a hard workout session or indoor cycle class. Now, when I read this quote, it gives me chills because I witnessed my husband's life at risk, and I know firsthand it is the truth. Fitness can save your life.

In my early days as a personal trainer and nutrition coach, I thought fitness was about looking good, fitting into clothing better, and feeling confident in a bikini. Over the years, as I've shared, I learned that these are all just the bonuses to living a healthier lifestyle.

At its core, being active is about improving our overall quality of life. It's important to build strength in our muscles and bones, care for our heart and lungs, and maintain a healthy body weight and energy level.

If we work at this now, we can live our life to its fullest rather than having to stay on the couch and watch others live it all around us. Exercising gives us the ability to live our golden years feeling golden. It's about longevity, and sometimes, as in my husband's case, it's even about setting yourself up for the best possible chance to survive.

Curve balls happen. This one, neither of us saw coming, but I am thankful that Graham was prepared to fight. Ironically, the very exercise bike that helped to save his life was also the one that contributed to him having to fight for it.

It was a holiday Monday, and I begged him to stay home. He had some equipment maintenance and odd jobs that needed to get done at the gym we ran, so instead of relaxing with me on our day off, he went in to work.

All I knew was that he had been planning on climbing the ladder to do some checks on our satellite that was up near the roof of the gym. He told me it wouldn't take long, and we would have the afternoon to relax together. He was wrong. Relaxing was the opposite of what we would end up doing that day.

Have you ever ignored that unsettling, something-doesn't-feel-good-about-this feeling? I really didn't want him to go. I *begged* him to stay home that day. I assured him the work would get done another time, and we could enjoy the day together instead. When he told me it would only be for a few hours, I had this feeling in my stomach that I just couldn't shake, but I ignored it. I covered it over with the logic that I was being clingy for wanting him to stay with me. In hindsight, I should have told him I had a bad feeling, and he shouldn't go. Instead, I didn't, and off he went.

He left that morning around ten-thirty. It was just after noon when the phone rang. All I remember is that Dana, a wonderful woman who was a member of our gym, was on the other end.

She told me, "I can't tell you why, but Graham is going to the hospital, and you need to meet him there. That's all I can say." I said, "Okay," and that was it. She hung up.

I listened to the dial tone for too long. I was so caught off guard. My mind jumped to him falling off a ladder and injuring his head or neck. I thought, *What if he has to be in a wheelchair for the rest of his life?* Or worse, *What if he doesn't live?* You're probably not surprised to hear me say that the worry reel set in fast. So did the adrenaline.

I frantically began searching for my car keys, which were in the same spot they always were. I stared at them sitting on the kitchen counter and knew when I saw them that I wasn't thinking clearly. I fought hard to keep fear, worry, and panic far enough away that I could function to drive safely to the hospital. I remember telling myself out loud, "Focus, get to the hospital."

My hand shook as I put the key in the ignition, and I could feel my heart beating so hard. As it raced, so did I; a ten-minute drive took me five. I arrived at the same time the ambulance did, pulled into a parking spot, and watched impatiently as they brought Graham out on a stretcher. I ran to his side.

He was slightly upright, holding his right arm, which was wrapped in bandages. I exhaled a massive sigh of relief, knowing it wasn't his head that was injured. I remember thinking, *It's just a broken arm, no big deal.* It hadn't registered yet that the ambulance wouldn't need to be on the scene if it was just a broken arm.

Then, as they wheeled him in, I saw it. The white dressing used to cover Graham's hand was now an awful shade of red. When I looked at his face, I was shocked to see that it was pale white. I asked him what had happened but didn't get a clear answer because he wasn't making sense. He was in the early phases of shock.

They wheeled him quickly into a room, and I ran beside him. I watched as the nurse gave him morphine for the pain. Then I watched hesitantly as she took the dressing off his hand. He gave me a very serious, slightly horrified stare to warn me not to look. I was far too curious to heed the warning.

Brace yourself. I certainly wish I would have. All four fingers on his right hand were gone. I could see bones and what can only be described as a horror scene. It was shocking. I don't think I will ever get the image out of my mind.

Despite the state of his hand, I was so thankful it wasn't something worse. I figured fingers were a minor thing compared to the head injury my worry had convinced me this was.

In most cases, this would have been minor. However, this was far from most cases. The hand injury was just the start of a terrifying week.

We left our tiny rural hospital via ambulance to London, a larger city centre that was a two-hour drive away. Graham needed surgery. Chris, one of our kind and brave gym members, had collected the remains of his fingers and put them in a bag of ice. The doctors hoped they could salvage the fingers by surgically reattaching them.

As we drove, I remember telling myself, *This is no big deal. He will have a quick surgery, and we will be back home in no time.* I also remember not believing myself. That feeling inside my stomach was still there and worse than ever. I couldn't seem to shake it.

During the ride, I tried to piece together what had happened. He tried hard to explain through the pain. He told me he was oiling the indoor cycle bikes, and the paper towel he was oiling the fly wheel with got caught and quickly pulled his hand through the gears. It happened so fast he couldn't prevent it. Forty-five pounds of pressure came down across his fingers and crushed them.

At first, he thought he had just broken his hand. That's what it felt like. But then he looked at his fingers on the floor and realized what had happened. As he pieced together how serious it all was, he quickly grabbed a paper towel and applied pressure to stop the bleeding.

He yelled to Chris and Dana for help, had them call 911, get the remains of his fingers on ice, and then he sat down and asked for a drink of water, at which point he says he realized he was going into shock. He remembered from his first-aid training that thirst was a sign of shock.

How he was even thinking of the signs of shock is beyond me, but Graham is a cool-under-pressure kind of guy. Me, on the other hand, let's just say it's good I wasn't there that day. Being alongside him in the ambulance and seeing his injury was hard enough on me. I know had I been there, he would have been picking me up off the floor.

The surgery was nine hours. Not all the fingers could be fixed. Two of them were reattached, and the others revised. I waited by a phone in a tiny waiting room at the hospital for what felt like forever.

I waited, and of course, I worried. My mind drifted to and from fear. I worried that he could die during surgery, and then I rationally reminded myself that it was just his fingers. I kept assuring myself with the logic that the whole thing was minor. And it was minor, but soon, it would become major.

It was two in the morning when I got the call from a nurse telling me Graham was out of surgery, and I could come in. I was so relieved to see him. He was sleepy but looked much better than he had in the ambulance. There was more colour in his face, and his very serious demeanor was replaced with a smile that looked like relief.

The nurse told me he would need rest and that I should get some, too. I knew she was right. There wasn't room for me to stay at the hospital, so I begrudgingly got a hotel. I badly wanted to be at his side, and it was extremely hard for me to leave him, but I was exhausted and needed a good night's sleep. My parents had arrived in the middle of the night to drive me to the hotel. They stayed with me the first night.

The next day, I visited Graham, and he seemed much better.

They needed to keep him for a few more days, but things were looking good. I spent the day with him, enjoyed dinner at his bedside, and then headed back to the hotel to sleep. This was a night I will never forget.

I didn't sleep that night. Despite my best efforts, I just couldn't settle myself down, and I couldn't figure out why. I tossed and turned. My heart raced. My mind raced faster. I worried; I wrestled with so much fear, and I prayed to calm the storm.

I recall looking at the alarm clock beside my bed and seeing one, then two, then three in the morning and still being wide awake. It was one of the worst nights I've ever had. Little did I know, this restless night was the night I almost lost the love of my life.

I've always believed that we are connected to one another through something greater than just a physical connection, but after this night, I know it with absolute certainty. I know I was aware on some level that Graham was in trouble, and my restless night was a symptom of that awareness.

It was six in the morning when I got the call from the nurse telling me Graham had had a rough night and was now in step-up care. I didn't know what that even meant, and she didn't get into any details.

I asked if I should come right away, and she said calmly, "No rush, love. Take your time. He's just fine now." The tone of her voice gave me no reason to rush, but I still couldn't shake the sinking feeling in my stomach. It was as though whatever I had been feeling all along was confirmed by her phone call. I knew there was a reason I hadn't slept all night and step up care affirmed all my worries.

I raced through breakfast, even though I had no appetite, and then I headed for the hospital as fast as I could. As I walked, I was aware of the extremely unsettled feeling in the pit of my stomach that still hadn't dissipated. I knew something wasn't right, but I didn't know what I was supposed to do about it.

When I arrived at the hospital and asked for my husband in step up care, I was told he was in the intensive care unit. I was confused and shocked. *Why had no one called me in the night if he was in intensive care? He was fine when I left, and now he's in intensive care. Didn't we just get through the crisis? Now, we were in another unexpected one that was obviously much more severe.*

I followed the nurse in to see him. There were wires and tubes running every which way. It looked like something out of a movie. A giant heating blanket was on top of his body, and he lay completely still under it. I asked the nurse what had happened. She told me they didn't know, but they were looking into it and would let me know as soon as they found out.

I sat by his bed and stared at him in absolute disbelief. He couldn't speak, but his facial expression was one I never wish to see on his face again. Terror. He looked afraid, and he was whiter than the first time I had seen him right after the accident.

Graham rarely gets concerned. The sky could be falling, and he would calmly say, "It's going to be okay." You may think that's an exaggeration, but for real, that's how he is. So, when I saw his face, I knew exactly how serious this whole thing was because he was definitely not looking like it was going to be okay.

A circle of seven doctors stood just beyond the curtain discussing Graham's chart. They didn't know I was at his side or that I could hear them, and I sat quietly to keep it that way.

One doctor said, "We gave the kid too much morphine." Another one spoke over him and said, "We don't know that for sure yet." There was tension amidst them and I could sense they, too, were very concerned and equally confused about what had happened.

Over the course of the next few hours, they concluded that he was severely overdosed on morphine. During the night, his lungs shut down. The doctors ran into his room with pads to help save him from a code blue. We still don't know if he actually died or if they arrived in time to prevent his heart from stopping. We still don't know a lot of details and likely never will.

What Graham remembers is that a nurse came in to give him a morphine pill because they wanted to wean him off the pump. He told her he didn't want the pill because he was feeling so nauseous. She insisted because the doctor had ordered it, so he listened. Thank God he did because what happened as a result is why he is still alive.

Within a half hour of taking the pill, he threw up, and though he remembers feeling completely out of it just before he got sick, he leaned over and hit the emergency button that called the nurse. Then he passed out, and his lungs stopped expanding.

Because he hit the button, the nurse came to check on him and could call a code blue and get him the help he needed. His body had received so much morphine that his lungs had stopped functioning.

It could have been a faulty morphine pump. It could have been the way his body metabolized the medication, or it could have been that he was simply given way too much. One doctor thought for sure they underestimated his size and gave him too large a dose.

What we knew for sure was that Graham was strong enough to make it through the next forty-eight hours. The doctors told him that his physical fitness level was a difference maker in his survival.

All that we have as any kind of explanation for what happened to Graham that night is an X-ray that shows the pads on his chest where they prepared to jump him, and his lungs filled with gray areas where no oxygen was present.

Over the course of the next twenty-four hours, I watched Graham fight to live. I remember staring at the heart rate monitor and being so concerned. It was as if he was running a marathon. His heart was beating over 190 beats per minute for hours while he sweat the morphine out under a heating blanket.

I remember watching his oxygen levels dip far too low and the nurse continually turning up the assisted oxygen so he could breathe easier. I remember asking her how long his heart could physically sustain that kind of speed. She told me that we are lucky he is in good shape, and because his heart was strong and conditioned to exercise and variance, he would be fine.

His heart and lungs were strong enough to endure this fight because he had trained at intensity regularly. He was prepared, and he didn't even know he had been preparing. Not everyone gets the opportunity to be ready. I'm so grateful that he was.

Much like my car accident, Graham will tell you this was his real moment with God. He says with absolute certainty there were more people in the room than were actually in the room. He remembers wondering if they were angels. He remembers feeling loved and safe and at peace, and he is certain there was Christian music playing in the room. To this day, he says he felt God was with him that night and believes God kept him alive.

I wasn't there, but there are a few things I know for sure. Graham and I are more connected than I ever realized because his scary night was a night I had to battle through, and something major happened that was life changing for Graham; faith became a part of his life in a much bigger way after that night, and the difference was noticeable. He believed deeper in his purpose. He was more grateful than ever to be alive, and he talked about God and heaven and faith more than he had in many years.

The experience gave us a whole new perspective and approach to our wellness career. Fitness and food matter. Living a healthy lifestyle is so much more important than looking good at the beach; it's about feeling good, being healthy, and being ready for whatever curve ball comes our way. Looking good is just the side bonus.

I recently had a conversation with Graham about how important it is that a spouse or a mom exercises. He had been in the thick of building another fitness facility, and his workouts were lacking. I'm extra sensitive about him missing workouts since this near-death experience, so I interrupted his focus one day with a loud declaration, "It's so important for you to exercise, not just for you but for all of us." He agreed and reluctantly took a break from work to move his body.

Afterward, he shared with me how true those words were. He told me how his mind felt clearer, and he was so much less stressed. He had more energy and came back from the gym feeling better for everyone and everything that needed him.

Exercise is like making a bank deposit. When you do it today, you're depositing strength, energy, mental clarity, and better health into your future. When you miss it today, you're withdrawing the same things.

I recognize it's not always as easy as simply reminding our loved ones to exercise, and then they do it. Many people struggle with making movement a regular part of their lives, myself included. I'm not always in the mood for it, and as much as I enjoy it, I'm human too and would often much rather relax instead. That said, I always feel better after having moved my body.

I tell my clients that it doesn't have to be big to be good. Every bit of movement we do counts. Ten minutes is better than zero. Running is fantastic, but walking is still movement and good for the body.

Because it is work, we sometimes prefer to avoid it, knowing full well it is the very thing we should do and need to do to be healthy, sleep better, de-stress, and live with more energy.

What we don't always see is that although getting a workout in is in fact work, it's also work to avoid exercise—future work, that is. When we sit on the couch instead or eat the better tasting, less healthy stuff, or have another glass of wine, or lounge around rather than move our bodies, it seems as if we are living in ease, but years from now, the cost is that our daily living will become the work.

Shoveling the driveway, gardening, carrying in groceries, even going for a walk, or climbing a flight of stairs will become harder than they once were. If we avoid the work today, we aren't saving ourselves from work; what we're doing is making easy things harder in the future and causing more work for ourselves in the long run. Every day, we choose whether our future will be easier or more difficult, even if we don't realize it.

We owe it to our loved ones to take care of our health, and that includes exercising regularly. When we neglect our bodies, we are missing out on the energy needed to give our best self to everyone who needs and loves us.

Our kids may pay the price for our sedentary lifestyle in the present and the future. I remember speaking with one of my busy mom clients who shared how she's much too exhausted to play with her kids at the end of the day. She often sits and watches them play instead.

I could see by the sad look in her eyes that she desperately wanted to be able to join them, and I know they wished for the same. Within six weeks of exercising and eating better, she was jumping on the trampoline and swimming in the lake by their home with them.

She had more energy to play with her kids. She was sleeping better and had life back in her eyes. Her husband had joined in on the workouts too, and the whole family was happier, healthier, and more energetic. Her kids got their mom and dad back.

It wasn't magic. They simply exercised four times a week for thirty minutes each time and chose healthier food options, within reason. She shared how she wasn't always motivated to do it, but the more she forced herself to simply do something, even if it was small, the better she felt. She was disciplined, and it paid off.

In the years to come, her children won't have to slow down for her to keep up with them; they'll likely have to speed up to keep up with her. And, as she ages, her body will continue to be strong and healthy, so rather than them needing to care for her, she'll be able to care for their kids—her grandkids.

Having discipline means we exercise whether we're in the mood to, whether we are too busy, and whether we have valid excuses or far-fetched ridiculous ones. There are people who need and love us. There are people who depend on us, and we need to do our part in staying healthy for them and for ourselves, and when we do, everybody wins.

This applies to every age, but especially as we age as parents, we owe it to our children to care for our bodies, so they don't have to do it for us. Obviously, some circumstances are out of our control as we age, but fitness isn't one of those things.

I never wish to burden my children with having to help me when and if I could have prevented needing that help. It's not fair to them, and that applies to spouses, too.

My children and I depend on my husband. It is one of his responsibilities to care for his body with fitness, healthy eating, taking his vitamins daily, and getting the sleep he needs to stay healthy and strong.

When I first start working with a mom, it's not uncommon for her to struggle with feelings of guilt for taking time away for herself to exercise. Moms place a lot of pressure on themselves to care for everyone else, and when it comes to caring for themselves, they would more often prefer to set their needs and wants aside and meet everyone else's instead.

When I explain to moms that it's selfish if they don't carve out time for themselves, they take a while to believe me. So many moms, myself included, have bought into the sacrificial lie that a good mom gives herself, and all of her time, away. A good mom cares for herself so she can be better for all those who need and love her.

As you know, I learned this the hard way, and I share my story so others can learn from my mistake and save themselves from making the same one. But before the meltdown I shared earlier, I had an opportunity to learn to care for myself, and it came in the form of another crisis.

A few years after Graham's accident, we had our first and second son, Andrew and Levi, and were thrown yet another curve ball. It was any mom's nightmare.

When my oldest son, Andrew, was three, he almost died. The week before he was hospitalized, I noticed he looked pale. That was it. There was nothing else out of character aside from being a little moody, which I attributed to lack of sleep and a typical three-year-old adjusting to his now-mobile younger brother.

Because of my experience with anemia, I simply thought his iron levels were low. I had a doctor's appointment booked for myself to check my iron, so I took him with me.

When the doctor saw him, he reassured me that we likely had nothing to worry about. Andrew was running around full of life and energy, climbing on the hospital bed and swiveling on the doctor's stool, just like his usual self. Our doctor ordered the blood work because he agreed Andrew looked very pale.

At 10 p.m., Graham got a call on his cell. It was a lab tech at the hospital telling us to get Andrew into emergency as fast as possible. She said he needed medical attention right away.

Graham, being the calm, uneasily shaken man that he is, asked the lab tech if she was certain we needed to wake Andrew up and take him to the hospital in the middle of a snowstorm. He was hoping it could wait until the morning, and so was I.

We were both hoping it wasn't as serious as it sounded. She insisted this was an emergency and that we needed to get Andrew help right away. His hemoglobin was at a 32, and he could die if we didn't move fast. The average healthy hemoglobin for a child is well over 100. She told us to get him in, or he may die.

Obviously, my heart sank as my mind went to all the worst-case scenarios. A few years before Andrew was born, I had almost lost Graham to his sudden accident. My heart was back to that moment, and my head told me this would be even worse. I was terrified.

We decided I would stay home with Levi, who was sleeping,

while Graham raced half-asleep Andrew up the road to our local hospital. We both hoped this was a false alarm. The doctor was in shock at the report of his hemoglobin levels and ran more bloodwork to be sure. The second report confirmed our fears; Andrew was in trouble. We were sent to the London Ontario Hospital for further investigation.

It was an hour's drive through a snowstorm, and Graham insisted he be the one to do the drive. Everything in me wanted to go with them and be there for Andrew, but by that point, it was midnight; the storm was even worse, and there was no way we could get childcare for Levi. I had to let them go.

As he packed things up to head to London, I will never forget Andrew's words. I leaned over to get him into the car seat and hugged him as tight as I could. I was trying hard to fight back tears because I didn't want him to worry. He then placed his hand on my arm and told me, "Don't worry, Mommy, God is with me, and I will be okay." Much like his dad, our Andrew has a way with words, and he brought me some calm in that very terrifying moment. Tears filled the corner of my eyes as I closed the van door.

I wanted to believe that as Graham had survived, Andrew would too. As I watched the van pull away, I was fighting hard to hang on to that hope. Standing in the freezing cold, watching snow circle around me, I stopped trying to be strong and broke down into inconsolable sobs. I felt alone and out of control. I begged for God to save my child.

I was desperate and wanted more than anything to go with him. I would meet them in the morning and, until then, wouldn't sleep a wink. A helpless, out-of-control feeling that was all too familiar flooded over me. Fear stole my thoughts and filled my body with adrenaline. Despite having faith in God and a firm belief that everything happens for a reason, the thought of losing my child shook my entire world. *What if he dies, and I never hug him again?*

The days ahead were exhausting. Lots of testing finally landed us in Oncology, and I feared the absolute worst. Thankfully, after many more tests, cancer was finally ruled out, and we were sent to the haematology specialist where we learned Andrew had a rare blood disorder called TEC (Transient Erythroblastopenia of Childhood). Essentially, something stopped his bone marrow from working, and he was slowly losing red blood cells. He was dying of oxygen deprivation.

Because of the lack of oxygen, his heart had developed a murmur to keep up. He had the lowest functional hemoglobin score any of the doctors had ever seen. He was still running around and seemed to have energy, even though his skin was now a pale yellow. The doctors speculated that Andrew's body had kept moving in an effort to keep his blood flow faster. They also told us his heart would have likely given out first. The body can only compensate for so long. We were very thankful Andrew's heart was as strong as it was because it was over pumping to keep him alive.

I remember calling everyone I know and posting on social media, asking for prayers for Andrew. The thought of not having him with us anymore was unbearable. As much as I wanted it to be in my control, I knew I wasn't. As I share this with you, I'm taken back to the intense shock, fear, and helplessness I felt as I witnessed my beautiful child endure needle after needle after needle.

I couldn't protect him from it, and I desperately wanted to. At the time he called them "pokeys." He would beg me, with his big green eyes and exhausted plea, "Please, no more pokeys, Mommy," to which I wanted to wrap my arms around him and promise him no more, but I couldn't make that promise. And that broke my heart.

As moms, we have this intense desire to protect our children. It's in our nature to want to prevent our children from experiencing any pain, sadness, failure, or grief. It's funny that our nature is to protect them, and yet, allowing them to fail and experience pain and sadness and the many challenges of life is how they learn and grow and appreciate the good things life offers. Sometimes, we need to let go.

Our nature is to bubble wrap our kids, and yet, bubble wrapping them isn't healthy for them. It protects us from having to witness them in pain but prevents them from learning and growing the way they need to. In those moments with Andrew, I couldn't do what I naturally wanted to do. All I could do was pray and be there to hold him while he navigated this new experience and showed us how tremendously brave he truly was.

Andrew needed blood transfusions to get more oxygen and blood into his body. They had to break them up into smaller amounts of transfusions so his heart wouldn't get overloaded and fail. The hope was that more blood would get Andrew's bone marrow working again and put this whole thing behind us.

As we waited by his bedside watching a blood donor's blood save his life and praying that Andrew wouldn't have any allergic reactions to the new blood, Graham looked at me with a deep concern. "You haven't slept for days, and I get that, but you also haven't eaten much. You need to eat, Alison."

Of course, he was right. It was then that I realized how hungry I was. It was also then that I had this amazing realization; I hadn't taken care of myself at all for four days straight—no sleep, very little food, barely any water, no shower, and constant worrying. It was awful. I was on a fast train to total derailment in the middle of our crisis. Had I kept going like this, I wouldn't be able to care for anyone; I would be the one needing to be cared for!

I realized that to be healthy for Andrew, taking care of myself was vital. It wasn't easy to leave his bedside to eat, rest, and shower. I feared taking one second away from him. My mind would race to thoughts like, *What if he dies, and I'm not there beside him?* I had to force myself past these fears and take this very important time so I could come back rested and much more levelheaded.

Graham and I worked as a team to ensure Andrew was getting everything he needed and so were we. Levi was in good hands with loved ones so we could focus our energy where it needed to be at that moment.

The great news is that the blood transfusions got Andrew's bone marrow working again, and he is now, as I write this, a happy and healthy, very energetic ten-year-old. I am so thankful that he is still with us. I am thankful for blood donors. I am thankful for great doctors, nurses, and personal support workers. I am thankful for all that the Ronald McDonald House does to help children and their families at the London Ontario hospital. I am thankful for all the prayers and support that kept coming from loved ones and even strangers during this intensely challenging time, and most of all, I am thankful to God for saving my son's life.

As much as I do not love to revisit the heart wrenching emotions these memories bring back, especially the awful feeling of helplessness that comes with being out of control of the situation, I love the reminder of what a blessing Graham and Andrew are in my life. On the hard days, that reminder allows me to be much more patient and appreciative of everyone I love.

The lessons these curve balls brought are some of the most valuable ones I've ever learned. When our children are sick or going through challenging times, we so quickly set ourselves aside, but we can't do this. We can't do this when they are sick, and we can't do this when they are healthy. We need to be a priority to be effective and healthy for everyone who needs and loves us.

Part of that means taking care of our physical body, not just preparing it so it can handle a crisis but also caring for it so our children learn healthier ways to cope with stress, worry, and life. When our kids see us exercising to de-stress and be healthier, they are far more likely to follow in our footsteps.

Any mom who has told their child a million times to clean up his or her room knows exactly what I'm talking about. We can tell them things hundreds of times, but showing them, with our actions, choices, and the way we live our lives, is a million times more powerful than any word we could ever speak.

When we exercise, we model to them how to care for their bodies, and we give them the tools they will need to stay healthy and strong as they become adults. We also give them an incredible tool that combats anxiety, overwhelm, stress, and depression better than any medication ever could.

When we exercise, we clear our minds, de-stress our brains, and increase blood flow and nutrients to our entire body. If we don't exercise, there are massive consequences to our mental, emotional, and physical health. If we don't exercise, we could be missing the chance to prepare for a crisis or opportunity we know nothing about.

The hard question is, are you prepared? We can't see the future. Life is full of curve balls. If a curve ball was thrown your way today, could you know with certainty you have given yourself the best possible fighting chance? If the answer is no, it's not too late.

Starting is the most challenging part, but if you start by placing meaning and a purpose behind it, it will give you the fuel to stick with it. What I mean is this; rather than simply deciding that exercise is a sweaty workout, instead decide that exercise is your life insurance policy.

We don't take exercise serious enough. We don't view it as a life-or-death necessity, but it is one. We need to realize that and make it a non-negotiable part of our lives. If we don't have our health, we can't enjoy any part of the life God has gifted us or serve him in the way he designed.

Many people view workouts as something they have to do, rather than something they get to do. We forget that the investments we make in our body today will impact our quality of life tomorrow. We forget how important it is to care for the one body we get to live in. It isn't selfish to take time away to exercise; it's selfish not to. Sometimes, we get that mixed up.

So, for all these reasons and so many more, exercise is one

of the pillars in my life necessary to not just overcome my worry struggle but to face whatever life as a busy mom throws at me and to ensure my health is good for myself and all those who depend on me today and tomorrow.

After a workout, I am calmer; any worries I have dissipate and are placed into a healthier perspective. I have more logic and less emotion once I've cleared my mind with a good sweat session, and I always walk away from it knowing that I just gave myself a fighting chance. Exercise can save our lives. Having this powerful meaning behind why I do what I do has allowed me to do it anyway, on the harder days, when motivation is low or not there at all.

As moms, our piles are full; I really can relate to that. Sometimes, responsibilities trump good intentions. On busy days, remember this: progress, not perfection. Move a little more today than yesterday; take smaller steps, but keep moving. Be kind to yourself, have patience and love for your body, and rather than trying to force it to look a certain way, move it so it will give you the energy you need to do all the tasks required of you. Your body deserves this kind of love.

We all have lumps and bumps, wrinkles, and stretch marks. Nobody is perfect. It's not about that. It's about this: to live fuller, with more energy, better health, and a clearer mind. The pile you're carrying needs to get set down, and you need to be picked up. Part of prioritizing yourself is caring for the one body you get; everything on your pile is lighter when you do this. You matter, too, mom, and your health truly is one of your greatest assets. I bid you to get moving.

Now, if I could change the quote a little, I would say it this way: "Train as if your life depends on it because every day it does." How you care for your body today matters today, and it matters tomorrow. Your health is valuable and every day your life depends on you caring for it. Choose to exercise not only because it melts the worries away but also because it gives you the strength to face whatever may come your way.

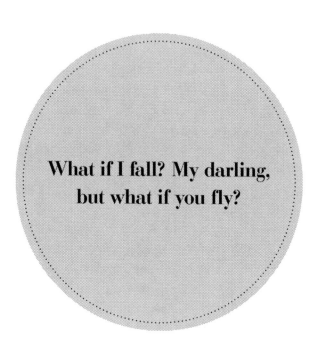

What if I fall? My darling,
but what if you fly?

CHAPTER 7

The Best is Yet to Come

I still struggle. Even though I have faith. Even though I have done, and continue to do, the inner work. Even though I eat real food and even though I exercise regularly.

God has provided me with the tools to live free from the exhaustion and stress of worry, and each step forward has brought me further from the struggle I used to face. However, challenges still arise, and sometimes, I still worry. Feeding a healthy fire has made a massive difference in my life, and I've made progress. Now, I struggle better.

I was reminded of how far I've come when I was in another car accident. This time, the car survived, but I didn't fare quite as well. I was in the passenger's seat, and we were at a stoplight. The person behind us didn't notice the red light and rear-ended our mini van. The hit was hard.

Thankfully, our kids weren't with us, but unfortunately, our fitness coaching team was. The good news is that most of the people in the vehicle were okay. The bad news is that not everyone was, myself included.

I placed my left arm on the dashboard to prevent my head from hitting it and injured my shoulder. That was the minor part. I knew I had a concussion within minutes of the accident. That was the part that set me back for months.

A few years before this accident, I was playing soccer and took a ball to the head so hard I was out for over a month with a concussion. This time was worse. I had horrible headaches. I kept forgetting where I put things. I couldn't focus on anything or anyone for longer than a minute, and I was anxious, frustrated, and struggling to stay positive.

The accident didn't just affect me; it rattled my entire family. With tears in his eyes, my middle son, Levi, exploded at me one night, "Mom, I already brushed my teeth. You asked me five times, and I told you all five times I already brushed my teeth. Stop asking me if I brushed my teeth!"

He was seven. He didn't quite comprehend that each time I had asked him if he brushed his teeth yet, I had forgotten about the time before. I felt absolutely awful. I completely understood his frustration. The feeling was mutual.

Head injuries are extremely difficult to navigate for everyone involved. Unlike a broken bone, no one can see them. On the surface, the person looks perfectly fine, even when they aren't.

For a while after the tooth brushing incident, I walked around sporting a band aid on my forehead. It was a reminder for my children to be a little quieter around me and a lot more patient with me. But honestly, it was just as much a reminder for me as it was for them.

Every time I looked in the mirror, I remembered to stop being so hard on myself, to slow down, to allow my brain the time it needed to heal, and to try to decrease my frustration with the whole thing.

All was going well with my recovery until one night I burned dinner and totally lost my cool with my kids. Emotional regulation can be a challenge on a good day for any mom. Throw a concussion on top of an already full pile, and it doesn't take much to tip it over.

My boys were hungry and getting under each other's skin. I don't remember what they did exactly, but I asked them calmly three times to be a little quieter. They did the exact opposite, and as they ramped up, the fire alarm went off. This concussion really affected my short-term memory and left me extra sensitive to noise, so the fire alarm was the tipping point.

As it blared in my ears, and the kids continued to add to the noise, the smell of burnt sweet potato fries flooded my kitchen. I could feel my blood pressure soar. My head throbbed, and instead of removing myself from the environment like I normally would have, and obviously needed to, I overreacted and yelled at the top of my frustrated lungs some words I shouldn't even write.

Confession, I'm not perfect. This was not my finest moment as a mom; that's for sure. It probably won't be my last imperfect moment, either. It's so good to be at a place where I can accept being human and know that I will make mistakes. My focus is on making progress and learning from the days I mess up. Perfection is no longer the goal.

Of course, I immediately regretted my meltdown, but I knew I couldn't take it back, so I soldiered on even though I wanted to crash. I waved a rag in front of the fire alarm, then moved into the kitchen to salvage a few fries. I felt a tug on the bottom of my shirt. My four-year-old looked up at me and repeated what I had just screamed.

When I heard the already painful words come out of his sweet mouth, the regret and guilt smashed into me like a heavy wave. I knelt down and looked into Zachary's beautiful eyes and apologized. He forgivingly reached his arms out and gave me the biggest, warmest hug. I could feel tears pooling at the corner of my eyes, and I knew the dam of emotion was about to break. I was frustrated and overwhelmed by this concussion, and I couldn't hold it in any longer.

I served dinner as quickly as I could, and while they ate, I crawled into my bed in hopes my head would stop throbbing. The tears came rolling down my face the second I hit the pillow, and as they did, I let the worry creep back into the corners of my mind.

Old habits have a way of sneaking up on us when we are weak

or presented with challenges. If we welcome the opportunities, they can be a chance to get stronger by embracing the fight through the temptations to slip back. But the fight is never an easy one, and I was losing.

Laying in a pile of frustrated tears with major guilt for yelling at my boys, I entertained the worry for a few minutes. I let myself go back to the darkness of this awful habit. *What if I spend the rest of my life asking the same questions over and over, not remembering where my keys are, or even where I'm supposed to be? Will I always be so out of control of my emotions? Will I forget to pick my kids up at school or show up for one of my clients or that dinner is in the oven? What if I'm left with permanent anxiety and memory loss? What if I will always be impatient with my children and even angry with them for no reason? What if I never get better?*

Isn't it funny how when everything is going well in our life, it's so much easier to be positive and live worry free? It's when all chaos is breaking loose that we're tested. When things are challenging, we shift back to our old default settings despite all the work we've done to overcome them. But this relapse was important. It allowed me to see just how far I've come because this time I struggled better.

Rather than spend hours going over all the what ifs or Googling long-term concussion outcomes, I fought back with a different focus. This took awareness, effort, and a lot of prayer. I had to know that the thoughts I was entertaining were not productive ones, and then I had to make a conscious choice that I would instead focus on something positive, and I had to pray and have faith that I would overcome this struggle.

I interrupted my worrying with the questions: *What if I am learning something from all of this? What if I'll come back from this stronger than ever before? What if all of this can teach me something valuable that I can then share with others? What if it all works out for the better?*

Aren't these way better what ifs? Celebrate with me a moment here, friend; this is massive progress! I started to ask good questions, and those questions allowed for positive answers. I also started to ask myself what I can do now to get better rather than focus on all the things I can't do now. Then, I did my best to control the things that I could control and let go of the things I couldn't. Letting go included forgiving myself for losing my cool with my kids, and it also included letting go of any negative what ifs.

Worry is a choice before it's a habit. It's difficult to choose not to go there but equally difficult is living your life constantly trying to control every outcome and worrying about the outcomes that will probably never even happen at all.

During my concussion recovery, the choice I had was to control what I could control, which was to prioritize my health. My kids needed me healthy and strong again. My clients needed the same. So did my husband, and so did I. To do that, I knew I needed to care for my health more than I ever have.

I decided from that point forward that I would choose to do whatever it took to get healthy. I sought concussion specialists. I went to physiotherapy, massage, and got chiropractic care. I never missed a workout. Did you know exercise is so important for the brain? It supplies it with oxygenated blood and repairs tissues. Just thirty minutes can and will keep your brain healthy.

Instead of researching all the bad possibilities and outcomes, I researched brain health and learned more about the nutrients I needed to improve my recovery. I supplemented with Vitamin D and Omega 3s to give my brain the nutrients it needed to heal.

I drank more water. I ate healthy foods to ensure I was getting what my body and brain needed to stay strong. I refused to let my frustration stoop me to the level of overindulging in sugary foods or alcohol that would just make me feel awful, and I practiced gratitude. Despite my frustration with how things were, there was still so much to be thankful for. There always is.

I had to make a conscious choice not to let my what ifs take me too far down the rabbit hole, so I focused on now rather than tomorrow. I let tomorrow worry for itself. I also had to decide how to view the accident. I had to decide that I would not go through this struggle without coming out of it better.

Sure, there were days I felt sorry for myself and wanted to throw a pity party, but those days were few and far between. Often, the choice to focus on what I can do today to get better helped pull me out of the pity party.

I firmly believe that everything that happens *to* us also happens *for* us—if we choose to let it. There is always something to gain from something hard. Since my concussion, I have been able to help others with theirs.

One woman was so comforted to know she wasn't alone in facing her concussion and hopeful to hear that I had made a full recovery. I could share all that I had learned and help her with her recovery process because of having gone through this. I would never have been able to reach my hand back and help encourage others had this not happened to me. There is good amidst the not so good.

Struggling better doesn't mean we don't struggle at all. I don't believe there is a magical moment when we've learned so much that the challenges stop coming. Life doesn't work that way.

Struggling better means we get back up quicker than we used to. It means we have more awareness than we did before. It means we know our triggers and can catch ourselves before we overreact or fall, sooner than we would have in the past. It also means we have access to more tools and know how to better navigate the challenges when they arise.

Struggling better for me means that I have chosen to ask myself better questions. Where I once asked, "Why me?" I now ask, "What can I get from this?" Where I once asked, "How can this be happening to me?" I now ask, "What can I learn now so I can I help others get through this in the future?"

What if you started asking yourself different questions all

together? Tony Robbins says, "The quality of your life comes down to the quality of the questions you ask yourself on a daily basis." He's right. Better questions bring better answers and can steer you in a positive direction, as opposed to a negative one.

What if you pondered what could go well instead of what could go wrong? Begin asking yourself, *What if things turn out amazing? What if the best is yet to come? What if there is something beautiful here for me to learn or experience? What if I succeed? What if I discover something I didn't know about myself? What if this trial can help others through theirs?*

David Goggins is a man who asked the right question at the right time, and if he can do this at rock bottom, anyone can. His story is so inspiring. His father was an abusive alcoholic. He grew up in constant fear and what he describes as "toxic stress." He was always trying to avoid abuse and suffered from crippling fear and anxiety.

Later in his life, weighing in at 300 pounds, he walked into the Navy Seals recruiter's office and asked to join. Every recruiter there said, "There's no way, man. You are 297 pounds, and you've got to lose so much weight so fast. You can't do it."

He had eight weeks and needed to lose at least one hundred pounds. He says that after hearing several recruiters tell him it would be entirely impossible, he remembers getting into his truck and asking himself, "But what if I could? What if I could pull off this miracle? How would I feel at the very end if I could defy all the odds?"

Instead of accepting what others said and walking away feeling foolish for ever thinking he could do it, he asked himself some amazing questions, and they were just what he needed to set his mind in the right direction. Because of this, his actions followed suit.

He lost over one hundred pounds in eight short weeks and became the thirty-sixth African American Navy Seal. A motivational talk he was doing caught my ear because not only did he ask the right questions, but he also thanked his mom for never helping him get back up when he fell.

He says the best thing she ever did was teach him to get up on his own. He explained, "She never picked me up. I would fail; I was at the bottom of the sewer, and she never picked me up. She never gave me that cookie and said, 'You know, son, it's gonna be okay.' Instead, she forced me to figure it out for myself. That's the biggest lesson that she taught me. I wouldn't be where I am today without that lesson."

I couldn't imagine not reaching out to help one of my sons when they needed it most. Moms are incredible helpers. We are so good at not only lending a hand but also intervening to prevent the fall. But our kids don't learn by having the world around them so safeguarded and cushioned that they never get hurt. They learn by the hard fall and the hard climb back up. Just like David Goggins's mom, we need to let them learn, and in doing so, we free them to live.

That freedom comes with letting go of our worry struggle. When we set it down and work to overcome it, we set the helicopter mom down with it, and when we stop stressing over what bad things could happen, we let them show us just how amazing they are at celebrating what is happening right now.

We can learn something valuable from his mother and from him. He had a choice when he got in his truck. He could have believed what the recruiters said to him, but he chose not to. He could have sat in the truck and sulked and beat himself up for hours because he got himself so overweight, but instead, he asked himself, "What if I can?" He made a choice to dream instead of sink, to believe instead of deciding to be hopeless, to take action instead of sitting in his inaction.

We all have the same choice as he did. We all have a struggle in front of us. His was his past and the weight he needed to lose. Mine was worry. Both could hold a person back if they chose to let it. Both can also propel a person forward. The difference maker is choosing to face the struggle head on, to look at it for all that it is, and to persevere despite it.

Unlike the worry wheel, which has you going around in circles, this positive focus propels you forward into new possibilities and unanswered questions that are waiting to be asked.

There are places you could go if you stopped holding yourself where you are. There are experiences and new opportunities you could have if you can be brave and make a choice to go for them, no matter what.

This habit is far more damaging than you even realize. It doesn't just prevent you from living your life; it has a massive and profound impact on your children and all those around you. In fact, you're holding back out of a fear of what could go wrong can and will prevent others from living their lives to the fullest. You could be holding yourself and others back by choosing to stay stuck with this habit.

Whenever I get focused on where I haven't gotten to yet, I like to look back to one moment in time where I'm reminded of how far I have come as a mother. It always gives me a good belly laugh and allows me to reflect and be thankful that I no longer parent from a place of fear. Scaredy Squirrel may have had some issues, but the old me had him beat.

If you're not familiar, Scaredy Squirrel is a children's book series, and the story I'm referring to is the beach day. The poor squirrel is so terrified of all the bad things that could happen if he goes to the beach that he goes to great lengths to bring the beach to his home so he can stay safe.

Beach day—when my fearless middle son, Levi, was three years old—was a day I will never forget. I was afraid he would drown, so I made sure he had a lifejacket on as he played in ankle deep water. He was beyond safe, but I had read somewhere that children can still drown in shallow water, and I had worried myself into believing the same could happen to him.

So, despite him being safe, I bubble wrapped him even more

just to be sure. His second layer of flotation protection was an inner tube that I had given him an excellent sales pitch about. "This is your magic floaty," I told him. He was easily persuaded. He wore water shoes in case he stepped on something sharp; there wasn't a rock in sight. He was slathered with sunscreen every hour on the hour. And I spent the entire day following around behind him wherever he went, exactly like a helicopter. Instead of us having fun together at the beach, I managed risks, and therefore, we didn't take any.

There I was, at a beautiful beach on a perfect day, not relaxing while I watched other moms read and suntan with their feet up while their kids played freely in the water. Instead of joining them, I let the fear and worry of the potential of what could go wrong steal my peace.

I never sat down once that day. In hindsight, I can laugh out loud about how ridiculous I must have looked, but at the time, it was all so real and serious. I was protecting my son from imminent death. This was no joke to me. I think Scaredy Squirrel and I would have gotten along wonderfully well that day.

Worry will keep us on the side lines, and that's what happened to me on our beach day. I came home from it completely exhausted. It wasn't fun or relaxing; it was work. That's what worry feels like—exhausting, stressful, muscle-aching work. We could have gone to the beach and had an absolute blast, but instead, I chose to worry.

I'm thankful this is no longer my parenting approach, but it stands as a perfect example of what could happen if we let worry control our lives. Some moms never make it to the beach at all. After sharing this story, one mom shared how she never goes in the water with her kids or lets them play in waves. Her fear of drowning is so real that it keeps her from ever getting into the water. I understand where she is coming from, but what I know now is that life is in the waves. Experiencing the adventure and fun of the water is true living.

So many moms are living their lives parenting from a place of worry and fear. They are constantly managing risks and stressing themselves out, trying to control the environment and mitigate danger. They focus only on potential risks and miss out on all the fun as a result. They don't live, and they don't let their kids live either.

The world is much the same. Playgrounds have taken away slides higher than six feet. Monkey bars are considered dangerous. Play structures have changed, and even the pavement I grew up bouncing off is now padded rubber or wood chipped to soften the landing.

Obviously, there's a balance, but if we never let our children take risks, climb a little higher, jump a little farther, or reach for that monkey bar, how will they ever develop a sense of independence or the wonderful feeling of accomplishment that comes from reaching the top? How will they acquire the lessons learned by trying again when they don't quite make it?

Choosing to set worry down has enabled me to be a much-less-stressed and more fun mom to my kids. It's allowed me to live again, to play, relax, experience adventure, and take risks I never would have taken, and to let my children take risks I never would have let them take.

Your worry for tomorrow is stealing so much joy, adventure, and peace from today. If you get too engrossed in trying to fend off what could happen, you'll wind up missing what is happening right now. You'll live your life holding yourself and your loved one's hostage to your fears. You'll miss the good things that could happen had you not worried so much about the bad things that likely never will.

I was so worried my children could drown that I kept them from leaving the shore. I was so worried they might get hurt in a tree that I refused to let them climb too high. I was so worried someone would take them that I never let them join in the fun of a crowd. I was so worried they would fall that I kept them from ever trying to walk. I was so worried they could die that I literally prevented them from living at all.

We bubble wrap them up in our selfish worries, and our bubble wrap becomes their prison. Our desire to prevent danger and control the outcome steals their success, independence, and peace.

In our efforts to cushion their world and prevent them from ever having to struggle, we steal their ability to learn and grow. It is in the struggle, the hard times, when life deals the biggest blows that they learn to cope, deal, problem solve, persevere, and get back up again. The struggle makes them stronger, brings them wisdom, and prepares them for their future in a way that only struggle can. The struggle is good.

If you were to help a butterfly out of its chrysalis, even with the best of intentions and the gentlest hand, the butterfly would likely die. As it struggles and works tirelessly to escape, it shuttles blood into its wings that it will need for the flight it's about to take. Without doing the work to get out on its own, it won't be prepared for the flight.

Witnessing someone we love struggling is one of the hardest things to go through, but we must understand that intervening to prevent it may not be the best approach.

How will our children gain strength and confidence in who they are if they never fall and, thus, never learn to get back up on their own? How will they learn to swim if we cling to them at the shore? How will they learn about danger if we never let them flirt with it? How will they learn boundaries if we never let them push them?

By interfering with all the best intentions to help our children avoid challenges, we are doing them a massive disservice. Their future self needs you to set your worries down and allow them the freedom to get themselves into challenges and then find their own way out. You're there if they need you but only if they need, not if they want you. Distinguishing that difference is important for kids and parents.

This isn't easy to put into practice, but it's important. It reminds me of the time Zachary went rollerblading. He was so excited to test out his new blades on a freshly paved road by my mom's house that he wore his helmet for the entire forty-five-minute car ride to get there.

As soon as we pulled into the driveway at Gramma's, he flew out the door and took off up the road. I ran alongside him. I knew there was a slight downgrade in the loop, and I warned him. I told him he needed to hold my hand when he got to that part, and he said he would.

Then, as the decline approached, and I reached out my hand, he refused. He wanted to be independent and race down it all by himself. I asked him a second time to hold my hand, and then I reached out and grabbed his hand in mine. I knew he would get hurt if he didn't allow me to help.

At the last minute, he ripped his hand away from mine, and as much as I wanted to chase after him, there was this moment of knowing that I needed to let him go.

Obviously, I knew the downgrade wouldn't be life threatening or anything severe, but it was still very hard to not chase after him. I knew he wouldn't learn by me running and forcing him to listen.

Sure enough, he gained too much speed, hit a bump, and fell onto his hands and knees. I ran to his side, and as he got up, I hugged him tightly. Right away, he apologized for not listening to me. Had I interfered, had I rescued him from that fall, he wouldn't have seen how important it is to listen to me when I ask him to.

My instinct was to chase after him and grab his hand, but that's not how he will learn. He needed the chance to flirt with danger and the opportunity to take a risk.

When he's a little older, we'll go back, and I will let him go down that slope without holding my hand, and he'll feel so accomplished when he does it. He won't be afraid to try it again, and I won't let my worry that he could fall prevent him from doing it.

Your worry can easily prevent them from ever facing a challenge, and when they do, because one day down the road they will, they will lack the ability to navigate their way out of the chrysalis. They will struggle with small things, and the big things will crush them entirely.

If you keep worrying and safeguarding their lives, your worries could become theirs. Eventually, they could absorb them and reflect them into the world and live out their lives cautious, fearful, and always holding back.

I'm not saying it's a guarantee, but it's possible they may live afraid. They may live nervous. They may live with unnecessary, preventable anxiety. They may live their lives clinging to the safety of the edge when it's the jump that teaches them how to fly. The jump is where real living happens, but if they are raised to fear it, the risk is going their whole life having never lived at all. Sadly, many people do this. They die without having lived.

The passing of my father was one of the most difficult challenges I have ever faced, but with it came the most beautiful gift of perspective. Knowing there was no cure for ALS and that he would die brought me a moment I won't soon forget.

The small stuff became smaller, and even the big stuff shrunk. It's the greatest gift because it's a chance to shift the way life has been lived. It's an opportunity to let the tiny stuff stay tiny—worry, fear, doubts, stress, the to-do lists—and let that small stuff take a back seat to what's important: faith, love, relationships, forgiveness, and gratitude.

My parents' lives are in boxes filled with photographs. All the memories and moments accumulate to make this beautiful life they lived. As I looked at all the photos, and we sat down to discuss funeral arrangements for my dad, I couldn't help but be grateful for my big moment—the one I walked away from forever changed.

I will cling to this painfully sad, heart-wrenching, beautiful gift that shifted all the complaining and worrying I've ever done into the most unimportant pile and reorganized everything that matters to me. It was the moment my dad held my hand and, with tears flowing down his face, tried to say goodbye, even though he could barely speak. As he closed his eyes on this world, I realized just how short life is. We're here today, and in the blink of an eye, our time on this earth is finished.

The sun is setting. Though we don't know when, we know it will happen. The fact is this; the sun will set for all of us, and if we can have this moment before the sky starts changing colors and before we see the end coming, we can have something valuable because it will change what the sun chooses to shine on and what it chooses to leave in the shadows.

We need to realize how fleeting life is before we see our final breaths approach. Otherwise, we will regret that we worried too much of it away and didn't live enough, and it will all be too late to change.

We will miss the beauty in this day if we are constantly focused on what could go wrong with it. We'll miss the potential tomorrow offers if we're only worried about what could go wrong.

When we think about all the things that moms carry, and we put them into perspective, we can see that they aren't all necessary. In fact, most aren't. Some can be set down for now; others can be set down for good, and others, such as our needs, as well as our beautiful children, should never be set down at all.

Worry can be set down. It doesn't have to be something you or your children or anyone else struggle with. Instead, it can be something you overcame. Like my beach day, it can become a distant memory of how you used to be. It can be replaced with how you are now—carefree, fearless, hopeful, and trusting that the best is yet to come. It truly is, but if you focus too much on what could go wrong, you'll miss what is going right.

Before I bring you to the end of worry and leave you with pages to ponder and hopefully a new beginning, I have one more story to share. I think it will give you a beautiful picture of the crossroads you may find yourself at and help nudge you in the direction toward freedom.

My youngest son, Zachary, got two slivers in his right foot at the same time. They were big, and they were deep. He was playing on some old deck boards in his bare feet and learned the hard way why shoes were invented. Graham and I arrived home from work to see him very upset about what had happened.

As he soaked his foot in warm water, he understandably fussed about wanting them out but not wanting to go through the painful process of having them taken out. He knew it would hurt.

Graham and I worked together to calm him down and then answered his many questions as he weighed his options and carefully considered the consequences. "If I keep them in," he pondered, "It will hurt to walk, but if I get them out, that will hurt too."

I watched as he came to realize that if he chose to keep them in, his biomechanics would have to be altered to work around the pain. He may not be able to jump on the trampoline the same way or run or bike or do any of the things he enjoys doing.

The longer they stay there, the worse things could get, and the potential for infection would increase as well. We were relieved that he came to terms with the fact that it would feel better to have the slivers out than it would for him to live with them in and in his words, "Walk on the side of his foot for the rest of his life."

After he soaked his foot, I held his hand while Graham used the tweezers to pry the slivers out. Zachy persevered through a lot of pain. We had to use a tiny pin to break the skin open, and we all exhaled a sigh of relief as Graham finally got a hold of the last stubborn one and pulled it out.

Worry is the sliver in your foot you may have been trying to live with. If you choose to keep it, you're making a choice that will affect your life. It will influence the way you walk, the choices you make, and the risks you take, or don't take. By keeping worry, you risk missing out on so many incredible opportunities.

Sure, it will be a process to get the sliver out. It may be challenging and even painful, but the relief that comes when it's finally gone is worth the effort needed to extract it from your life forever.

Faith, inner work, real food, and exercise are your tweezers. Bit by bit, your worrying habit will be removed and replaced with the freedom that can only be understood once you've had a stubborn sliver removed.

You need to let it go. It's a choice. It's difficult, but it is so much easier than staying in constant worry. Choose to work at getting it out of your life rather than work at keeping it in it. What we don't realize is that both require effort, but only one steals our joy.

Walk away from worry once and for all. Pull it out of your foot, throw it off your back, and instead, march forward with hope and peace. They're so much lighter.

The best is yet to come, and you don't even have to believe it just yet for it to be true. Simply decide that herein ends your constant worrying and turn the page to a new beginning.

Helping one person might not change the world, but it could change the world for one person.

CHAPTER 8

Strike a Match

Just days before I submitted the manuscript for this book to the publisher, I struggled with the last chapter. I wanted the book to have seven chapters, and I was determined to stick to this plan. The number seven represents completion, so I had decided that would be just the right number of chapters. I like completion.

I love the significance God places on numbers. They all have meaning and a purpose for him. In six days, God created the world and all that is in it, and on the seventh day, he rested because his incredible work was finished.

Regardless of how I tried to pare things down and move things around, chapter seven was too long. I was going to have to shorten it significantly if I wanted to stick to my plan, which I very much did.

I sent the chapter to some loved ones for their feedback, and as I waited to hear back from them, something interesting happened. God made a new plan.

I was teaching a barbells class at the studio my husband and I run, when one attendee, also a wonderful coach of ours, noticed the rep scheme of the workout I had designed were all sets and reps of eights.

She mentioned it aloud to me and shared how the class that she had led earlier that day was also all sets and reps of eights.

"Eight must be the number of the day," I told her, and then I shared the meaning of the number eight with her.

I had just read about David being anointed by the prophet Samuel to be King over Israel. David was the eighth son of Jesse. The writer shared how eight is the number that represents new beginnings, so I passed that on, and for a second, I wondered with excitement what new beginnings may be coming for her.

Thinking nothing more of it, I carried on with the class. Unbeknownst to me, God was speaking, but I wouldn't discover it until the next day.

Without having ever spoken to one another, both of my loved ones came back and told me the same thing about chapter seven. It doesn't need to be pared down, it just needs to be made into an additional chapter in the book—an eighth chapter. "Eight is a great number," one friend told me.

I immediately remembered the brief chat about the number eight in my class the day before, and as the memory came back, the hair on the back of my neck stood up in a good way. I knew it was confirmation that there needed to be eight chapters rather than seven.

Thus, here we are. Inspiration came in the middle of the night as I lied in bed wide awake, not worrying but writing this chapter in my head. I was comfortable. I had found just the right indent in my pillow. The blankets were in the perfect place. The temperature wasn't too hot or too cold, but just right, but I could feel the intense pull to get up and write.

Sometimes, we get set in our ways, and God speaks to us to let us know that He has a better way. What I know for sure is that this new worry-free life you and I can live is a new beginning. It's a fresh start at living life rather than avoiding it.

Just as I had to be willing to let go of what I wanted and had planned to make room for a different possibility, you'll need to let go of this habit to make room for a new way of living—one that

God has designed for you. One that is better than what you had planned for yourself. You'll need to set down fear and anxiety and the worry that is too heavy to carry, and in doing so, you'll allow the space for something new and good. This eighth chapter in your life is a fresh start. It's a chance to reconsider all of your old plans and perhaps venture to the edge of something new and exciting.

God's plans are always far better than we could imagine. He wants us to live an abundant, worry-free life, and if we let him build this eighth chapter when we thought we were finished at seven, he'll show us that seven wasn't good enough for us. The worry is finished. You've turned a new page. There is so much more to your life than living confined to seven chapters. There's an eighth one that's even better than you could ask for or think of, and if you're willing to embrace it, it can be an amazing new beginning for you.

The title of this book came at a time I least expected it. I was sitting on the very bathroom floor I had sat on during my epic mommy meltdown. This time, though, I wasn't melting down; I was helping another mom through hers.

I escaped to the bathroom to get a quiet, kid free space for five minutes so I could give her my undivided, uninterrupted attention. Shamelessly, I was hiding in the bathroom from my children. From time to time, I still do. It seems to be the one place they will not venture, thankfully.

My friend had called to chat because she was struggling with some things after having her second child. Like any mom with a newborn, she was tired. She was working to get her body back in shape after the pregnancy, trying hard to keep her marriage happy, and tirelessly juggling all the things moms try so hard to carry. On top of that, she was also battling post partum depression.

After deciding to seek help and get the medication needed to get her back on her feet, she was starting to feel a little more like herself but was worried about a lot of things and began to share them with me.

As I heard her ask what if repeatedly and listened to her list all the things she was concerned about, I heard God speak to me. It wasn't an audible voice that came roaring through my ceiling, but it may as well have been because it was so clear and deep within my soul that I knew it was the voice of God. I still know to this day that it was.

He said, "Don't let *what if* ruin *what is*." I was in the thick of writing my first book, and much like we do during childbirth, I had vowed to never write another book again. It was a daunting task, and I felt overwhelmed by the process and determined to never embrace another one like it.

Despite my plans, I knew at that moment that I had just been given the title to my second book. I can't explain how I knew it; that's faith, unexplainable but so real that the knowing within me couldn't be taken away or rationalized. I just knew.

I shared with my friend the words I had heard and hoped they would help her understand that, though her worries were valid, they could be stealing her focus away from the good she had in her life. If she continued to look at all the what ifs, she would lose focus on what is most important.

I am not the fixer; God is. I was thankful He provided me the words to speak to my friend and amazed how He could give us both the words we needed for our situations at the same time.

Then, I tucked those words away in my journal and honestly tried to take their advice myself. Sometimes, the advice we give others is also the advice we need, and as you've discovered, I needed that advice too.

Before I could ever get to a place of helping others, I needed to first overcome worry in my life. Thus began my journey to worry less and live more and my deep dive into the faith and inner work that needed to be expanded, along with a healthy focus on real food and regular exercise.

Fire—it can be destructive or productive depending on which one we choose to feed. I hope the matches in my hand have kindled a new fire for you. One that burns so brightly it allows you to see the endless possibilities that lay in front of you, the ones you deserve to have. Fan this new fire, mom. Keep it burning strong and let it change your life.

Focus on growing your faith, letting God show you the inner work that needs to be done, and caring for the one body you've been given with real food and regular exercise because there truly is a better way to live and a better way to be a mom. It doesn't have to be an exhausting experience. It can be a peaceful and joyful one.

Once this healthy fire is blazing, do me one favor; allow it to kindle a fire in the lives of other moms who worry, too. Together, we can put the entire habit out and ignite a healthier one.

I wrote this book because I don't believe the freedom that I've experienced was ever meant to be kept to myself. Nothing good should be hidden if it could help someone else. Our struggles can be other people's road maps through their struggles if we are willing to be open and reach our hand back. We need to let our freedom be contagious rather than keep it all to ourselves.

I was reminded of the importance of reaching a hand back to help others when we went for a family bike ride. We started out together but ended up getting split up along the way because Zachary had just mastered a two-wheeler and was moving a little slower. Graham stayed back with him to ensure he was safe, and I went ahead to check on Levi and Andrew.

Levi tends to be my most competitive child and is also very athletic. He had zoomed ahead of all of us to ensure he finished first. As I approached the finish line, I had this nudge to remind him how winners should behave.

As I thought about what I was going to say to him, I realized just how important it is to teach our children to win with integrity and love, and humbly encourage those who didn't win. Learning to lose and win is important.

I knew my youngest was determined to do the entire five kilometers, and I knew he was tired and still learning and needed the encouragement that meant so much more coming from his older brother than it did coming from his mom.

I also knew that Levi needed the reminder that winners don't just cross the finish line, win, and walk away. True winners cheer on the next in line. They pay it forward. I wanted him to know that winners reach their hand back.

As I got closer, I asked him, "What do winners do?" He looked confused at first, but I could see that he was pondering the question. Before he could answer, I let him know, "They cheer everyone else on."

His response made me proud, "I always do, Mom." And he's right; he really does.

I asked him if he would go back and cheer on his little brother. As I spoke, I was reminded of the time Jesus told Peter, "I have prayed for you that your faith would not fail. When you have turned back, strengthen your brethren."

This principle can be applied in so many arenas; when you've been helped, help. When you've reached the top, reach a hand back. When someone has encouraged you, encourage someone else who needs it, too. It's only when we open our hands that God can multiply the impact. Good things were never meant to be held in a closed fist. I don't believe he wants us to overcome our struggles and then never share with others to help them overcome theirs.

In the story with Peter, first Peter needed to be strong enough to strengthen his fellow disciples. He needed to learn to face and overcome his struggles, and that meant he needed to go through them first.

Jesus prayed he would overcome, and because of that, he did and was then able and equipped to reach his hand back and offer his brothers what they needed to return to the faith and begin the church.

Victory doesn't stop with us; it starts with us. It's not meant to be kept for us but also given away to help others succeed, too. True winners help others win and make them feel like winners by strengthening and encouraging them as they cross the finish line.

Zachary was tired as he biked up the road toward our home, but he finished with the biggest ear-to-ear grin as he heard us clapping and cheering for him. Everyone smiles bigger when they know they're being cheered for.

I'm cheering for you. I'm hopeful that you can set some things down that you've been carrying for too long and free yourself and your children from the weight and stress of living life on the side lines.

My hope is that every worrier mom can overcome this struggle and light some matches for fellow moms who are going through the same thing. We could all use a cheering squad and a little extra help.

Here's the good news; this is only the messy middle. There's more to your story. It's not the end yet, so you're not there yet. But I promise you this, you will get there, and by there, I mean to that beautiful place of progress where you can look back and be amazed by how far you've come.

But in the middle, it's messy, and that's okay. Things weave together nicely at the end. All the loose ends get tied up, missing links get reconnected, and there is clarity and understanding. Don't rush to that part, though; there is learning to do in the middle.

I recently heard a preacher speak about a boy who had a very messy middle. The story goes like this: He was five when his father, Jonathon, and grandfather, King Saul, were killed in battle. In a panic, his caretaker scooped him up to flee in fear he would be killed. In her haste, she dropped him, and both of his feet were paralyzed.

When he was older, King David learned he was alive and had flown to stay with Ziba. David wanted to show God's kindness to the boy and bring honor to his father, Jonathon, whom David loved, so he called for him to be brought to the palace.

He gave him all the land Saul had owned and provided workers for the land and invited him to eat at King David's table in the palace. The love of God covered him through King David, and he was overwhelmed by it. He bowed down and said, "What is your servant that you should notice a dead dog like me?"

But that's exactly what God's love did for us. He looked at a dead dog and restored it to life, and not just that, He made a seat at his table for us to eat with him. How awesome is that?

As I thought about how beautiful this story is, I also thought about the messy part in the middle where the boy lost his father, grandfather, his home, and the use of his legs all in one day. How horrible!

I thought of the trauma of being dropped by someone who was well meaning and whom he trusted. I thought about how he was living his life in hiding and fear, worried that he may soon be the next one killed. In one moment, his life had changed so dramatically for the worse, and the mess of it all was hard to see beyond.

If someone were to come and tell him that the best was yet to come, that he didn't have to fear or worry, that King David would restore all the land back to him and ensure he is fully taken care of, it may have been difficult for him to believe them, even though it was the truth.

It was then that I heard God say, "You cannot judge your story by the mess in the middle child. You will be restored in my time. It may not happen as fast as you would like it to. But it will happen because I am the God of love, restoration, and happy endings."

You may look at the messy middle and think it's the end, but the good news is that it's not the end at all. It's only the middle. There is more to come, and the more to come is good. In fact, God promises, "Though your beginning was small, yet your latter end would increase abundantly." (Job 8:7) So, I would venture to say that what is to come for you is great.

You may be down, but you're not out. It may look over, but it's only the middle, and the best part is up ahead. There is something to learn from the struggle. If you embrace it, it will change you for the better and give you the tools you'll need to not only help others but also face the next challenge wiser and stronger. If you fix your eyes on how awful and messy it all looks and worry about what else could go wrong, you may miss what is about to go right.

It may feel like it's all crashing down around you, but it's only for a time; the end isn't here just yet. Set down all the heavy things you're walking around carrying and take your eyes off the messy middle.

Let your faith rest in knowing there is more you haven't seen yet and be brave enough to dream that it's going to be amazing. Trust that his timing is perfect, and he will finish this well. You will see his hand in your life, and glory will come out of it.

The problem, the mess, the heap of all the stuff that seems so big, the fear, anxiety, doubt, and giant pile of worry, the to-dos, and burdens that accumulate, the struggles—none of this is too big for God, and it's not the end until he says it is. So long as there is breath in your lungs, it's only the middle. "All books are messy in the middle, child. Keep reading."

Your chapter eight can be the very best one for you, but if you let your mind spin out of control over the worst-case scenarios, you will never get a chance to live out or imagine the best ones. I want you to know that you can break this habit and take back your life from this day forward. Pray that you, too, can be set free, and I am certain God will answer that prayer.

You deserve to ask what if and have the answer that comes to your mind be a positive one. You deserve to be worry free, and the only way you're going to get there is by choosing to stop living with it and start living free from it.

This is a choice you'll need to make today and every single day, and as you do, it'll get easier, and you'll get farther away from the worrying mom you used to be and closer to the mom who lives more.

What if it didn't happen the way you feared but the way you hoped? What if you were brave and decided even if? What if the best was yet to come, and it was just waiting for you to stop holding back from life and simply take the first brave step?

It's time to enjoy what is. It's time to let what is be all that it was meant to be, and when you do, you'll soon see the life God wanted you to have when you became mom was a life filled with so much more peace and joy than you ever hoped or imagined.

It's a life where what if is dreaming instead of worrying, and the worry that once restricted your living becomes a distant memory, a memory of a sliver you once removed from your foot. And ever since, you can run pain free toward a life filled with peace, joy, hope, freedom, love, patience, and a faith that what lies ahead will be even better than your wildest, worry-free dreams.

As I leave you, I challenge you: If you're ever going to ask what if again, let it be to dream rather than to worry. Dreams create memories; worries create regret. You deserve the most beautiful memories, and all you must do is choose to dream instead.

Dream big, mom, because you were not made for small. The only thing small that you were made for was your beautiful child(ren), and as they get bigger, their lives will get better because you chose to live yours unapologetically, worry free.

"For I know the plans I have for you," declares the LORD, "plans to prosper you and not to harm you, plans to give you hope and a future."
–Jeremiah 29:11

Acknowledgments

Graham Brown – After sixteen years of marriage, I still have a crush on you. It has been a challenging ride at times but one I wouldn't want to do with anyone else. Thank you for your unmatchable, immovable support as I pursue all the dreams God has given to me. You've believed in me even when I didn't, and I love you and each of our three precious boys beyond words.

Lorraine Wells – Mom, thank you for being a brave trailblazer willing to try something new and scary. You're the reason I can do the same. You showed me how a mom can change the course of her children's lives for the better. Your journey helped begin mine, and I am forever thankful for all you are. I love you beyond words.

Megan Fish – Your gift of art to this world is an absolutely beautiful one. Thank you for your contribution to the cover and for the color and life you add to this world. It is a blessing to know you. (Check her out at https://paintingwithmegan.art)

Laura Eby – Thank you for restoring my faith in neighbors and friends. You are a blessing in my life, and I appreciate your support in this process, your delicious meals when I didn't want to cook, your willingness to listen, and the ease you bring with your presence.

Donna Mitchell– Thank you for your support, encouragement, feedback, and help with getting this book finished. I know you've been in the background praying, encouraging, and cheering me on, and it means more than I could express. You are a wonderful woman, and I am blessed to know you.

Douglas Baker – Thank you for always being willing to listen and for offering advice, support, and encouragement when I've needed it most. Your spiritual guidance has been a force for positive change in my life, and I am so thankful for you and your family and all you contribute to me and mine.

Ross Gilbert, Crossways to Life – Thank you for facilitating such a beautiful healing program. Your discipleship is a blessing in my life and the lives of many others, and I'm so grateful for you, for all you offer, for your colleagues, for the beautiful ELAT group that came together in 2022 (for Karen for telling me to "Just do it!"), and for a counseling centre that truly is making a difference. www.crosswaystolife.org

Jan Pritchard – You've seen and heard me, and it is because of that I can embrace being seen and heard. Thank you for showing me who I am in Christ, for challenging me to consider how deep His love truly is for me, and then helping me embrace the deep waters He has called me into with the faith that I can trust Him when I get there. You are a gift and a blessing in my life.

Printed in the United States
by Baker & Taylor Publisher Services